THE JOY OF HOMEOPATHY

THE JOY OF HOMEOPATHY

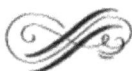

*Told through
real life stories*

EM COLLEY

Bold Fish Publishing

THE JOY OF HOMEOPATHY: TOLD THROUGH REAL LIFE STORIES

Cover design: Lel Nicholson Grindrod
Cover photos: Em Colley
Family picture: Laura Byrne
Medicine bottles: stock.adobe.com
Plant sketches in Stories 1-9: Enya Marczak
Animal sketches in Introduction and Stories 10: Olivia Marczak (Bright Eyed Artistry)

Edited by Helen Strong and Julie Trager
Published by Bold Fish Publishing
www.boldfish.pub

For my grandparents Dennis and Emmie Cowgill

your ability to see the joy and wonder in everyday things inspired and continues to inspire me.

PRAISE FOR THE JOY OF HOMEOPATHY

A perfect book to read for those that are interested in homeopathy in practice. The title reflects the author's passion for homeopathy, which comes from years of experience and witnessing the healing in both humans and animals. A 'Joy' to read!
Gill Graham, MFHom (Int), Vice President, Faculty of Homeopathy

The Joy of Homeopathy *is packed with stories from a dynamic homeopath's life—stories to enlighten the reader about the breadth and depth of homeopathy and about the potential for healing that's possible with this lovely modality. This little guidebook is full of inspiration. Oh and joy!*
Miranda Castro, FSHom, Homeopath, Author, Educator

Em has crafted a captivating book on homeopathy, presenting the elegant science through her eyes and clinical experience. She intricately blends concepts, history, statistics, critical analysis, meta-analysis and, most importantly, the diverse experiences of patients and homeopaths from around the globe. Delving into this book will inspire the

inquisitive mind to leap forward in the world of homeopathy.
Dr. Bhawisha Joshi M.D. (Hom) & Dr. Shachindra Joshi M.D.
(Hom)

Reading Emma Colley's The Joy of Homeopathy *was a great plea-sure—indeed, a great joy. From her many years of experience in homeopathic practice, Em has crafted a homeopathic gem, which happily fills the gap between professional works and self-help books for the public. It provides ideal reading for anyone interested in understanding the principles upon which homeopathy is based and, through charmingly-presented anecdotes, affords rich insight into what a wonderful friend this gentle, yet powerful, healing modality can be in family life. The book also gifts the practitioner an engaging and instructive text to be recommended to clients desiring to know more about the unique, individualising methodology of homeopathic prescribing.*
Dr David Lilley, past-dean of the South African Faculty of Home-opathy

In this book Em shows the process of healing with homoeopathy beau-tifully through stories that are relatable and authentic. A must for anyone who wants to understand what a curative journey may look like, or to delve deeper into a homoeopathic healing journey.
Camilla Sherr, FSHom, PCH

This gorgeous piece of work showcases Em's unwavering dedication and passion for homeopathy. I was inspired as I read about her remarkable successes in clinic and the profound impact she's had on people's lives. Homeopathy, as a beautiful system of medicine, is brought to life through Em's work, which she has fully embodied in this book. Her commitment and achievements are nothing short of extraordinary.
Haroula Battista, Dean of The Ontario College of Homeopathic Medicine

The remarkable stories of people on their journeys from illness to health are magical. We understand why they are ill! This is a clear exposition of the huge potential of homeopathy, beautifully written. Read this book at your peril. You won't only want to use homeopathy, but become a homeopath.
Geoff Johnson, VetMB, MA, MRCVS, RSHom, VetFFHOM, PCH

A wonderful read to understand why millions of people across the world use and trust homeopathy. Em's detailed cases from her clinic and personal experience bring to life with warmth, care and charisma how useful homeopathy can be in managing our health.
Cristal Skaling-Klopstock, MBA, FFHom(Hon), FSHom(Hon)

A positive, re-affirming book told through patient stories which delves into homeopathy and its life-changing potential.
Andrene Mills, RSHom, Principal of NWCH

A perfect introduction to homeopathy written with generosity and joy. Reminds me of the joy of reading Dorothy Shepherd before I then had to train as a homeopath!
Elaine Watson, Homeopath

Em's open minded and open hearted approach to empowering and supporting her patients is on full display in this gem of a book. Gently and respectfully she invites us to witness the power and scope of homeopathic medicine by sharing the stories of her patients. I wish I'd had this book available to me when I was in practice.
Sue Asquith, Retired Homeopath

A beautiful resource for those who are new to or curious about homeopathy and are interested in understanding the magic, not only of the pills but of the way in which a skilled and passionate practitioner works. Em writes effortlessly and elegantly about homeopathy because she lives and breathes it. I will be recommending this book to

my own clients to deepen their learning about this incredible holistic healing modality.
Nicola Corcoran, Naturopath

Em's book brings homeopathy to life in a way that's palatable, relatable and inspiring. I was left with a strong curiosity as to what it could do to help transform both my own health and that of my loved ones.
Georgina Marczak, Energy Healer, Reiki Master and Ayurveda Practitioner

This beautiful little book is a very elegantly written introduction to the wonders of homeopathy. The cases are clear, informative and accessible, and let the process live for the reader. Em has a real enthusiasm and passion for her work and every page brims with joy. This will now be my go-to book to lend or recommend to people who would like to get an idea of what homeopathic treatment entails, to see if they would like to try it for themselves. Thank you Em!
Bev Nickolls, Homeopath

Rarely was there such an apt title—the joy shines through, not only of the people Em has worked with but also in the explanations about homeopathy—not an easy thing to convey but Em does it brilliantly.
Sato Liu

The Joy of Homeopathy *is a joy to read. Em has a natural, engaging writing style as she opens up the fascinating world of homeopathy to all. I would thoroughly recommend this book, both to those familiar with homeopathy and its uses and to those who merely have a curiosity to learn.*
Josie Powley

This book covers what conventional medicine doesn't know about our bodies and minds. And it does it so well.
Natasha Serafimovska, Writer and Consultant

By skilfully interweaving the fundamental principles of homeopathy together with the very real-life experience of her patients, Em takes us on a compelling, often moving, journey of discovery. And if anyone was wondering whether it was worth trying homeopathy for themselves, just read what Em's patients have to say about their decision!
Karin Mont

The Joy of Homeopathy *gives readers an insight into the magic and mystery of this alternative practice of healthcare and healing. Using real-life case studies, it is a beautiful and powerful aid for anyone interested in learning about homeopathy and the benefits it can have on our health and well-being.*
Jen Armstrong, Professional Musician and Singer Songwriter

Disclaimer

This book is in no way intended to diagnose or suggest treatment for any of the conditions mentioned. The cases described herein provide examples of how homeopathy may be of help when homeopathic medicines are chosen according to the specific requirements of the person receiving the treatment.

Homeopathic medicines are prescribed for the individual, so whilst you may experience some of the symptoms described in the examples given, it doesn't mean the medicine prescribed in that particular case will be the right one for you.

Some of the stories will illustrate how the same homeopathic medicine can be used for more than one condition. But equally, two people with the same condition, for example eczema, could be given an entirely different medicine, based on their individual symptoms and personalities.

To me, it is important that everyone should have the best support for their health and well-being, whether that be from a strictly conventional medical model and/or a complementary therapy such as homeopathy. As you will learn in these pages, I am a great advocate of an integrated approach to health care and I always recommend that clients continue to work with their conventional medical team alongside homeopathic interventions.

CONTENTS

Introduction

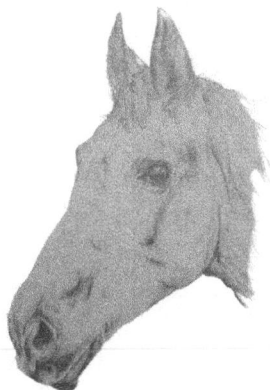

Kara—short for Karavana—was a stunning 16.3 hands[1] Czech warmblood, nicknamed 'the blonde bombshell' by a friend. A striking palomino mare, she was feisty at times and a wonderful trekking companion. We would ride for miles together along country lanes and several times we visited the Yorkshire coast on three-day trips, staying along the way at farms and B&Bs with stabling facilities. As a teenager, not quite sure where I fitted in the world, having these quiet, reflective times hanging out with our horse was a godsend.

When I was fifteen, Kara contracted recurrent uveitis, a rare condition involving inflammation of the eye that can cause redness, pain and even loss of vision. We were told by our vet that the condition was incurable and for some time, we gave Kara the recommended conventional treatment—regular steroid injections into her eyelid (which required sedation to administer) and daily anti-inflammatory medication. Blood tests showed that her liver was not tolerating the medications well, and in order to avoid having to use them to keep the uveitis at bay, our vet suggested removing her eye as a possible option. While surgery (and no longer having the eye) might have eradicated the disease, my parents decided to explore alternative solutions before they made that decision. I can see why the concept makes sense—remove the diseased eye, the disease is removed. But it didn't feel the right route to go down at that point in time; what if there was a less drastic solution?

My mum contacted a herbal company to ask if they could recommend anything. They referred us to Chris Day, a homeopathic vet and, frankly, something of a pioneer and champion of his time. Chris referred us to his equally brilliant colleague John Saxton, who lived more locally to us, and so began our first encounter with homeopathy. A few days after the initial consultation, we received the homeopathic pills, which we would stuff inside a piece of carrot to ensure Kara took them.

This next bit still makes me smile and I always imagine it like the climax of a film. The livery yard where she was stabled, located a mile up a fairly steep hill, became inaccessible by car due to heavy snow. My dad—the hero of this part of the tale—trekked up the hill, at times with swirling gales of snow whipping around him, once a day for five days to administer the tablets to our horse.

And just like that, Kara's eye disease went away. Even though our conventional vet told us it would just be in remission because it was incurable, Kara never had the disease again for the rest of her life. Cured, or incurable and in remission, Kara lived happily with two eyes for another fifteen years after those five tablets—no further steroid injections, no further anti-inflammatories and no further pain.

Years later, I met John Saxton at a conference and was able to thank him in person for his outstanding care many years earlier. I asked him if he could remember what he gave Kara. He couldn't recall, and the records had been shredded long before, so I'll never know which medicine gave me my initial experience with homeopathic treatment. It doesn't really matter... by any standards, the treatment was hugely successful. I wish I could say the experience convinced me to study homeopathy there and then but at the time, it was just something that happened. I had no idea it would lead me to where I am today. In any case, I remain grateful to all the people who played their part in the chain of events that was my first encounter with the wonderful world of homeopathy.

My intention in writing this book is to help you gain a greater understanding of homeopathy and what it can achieve. Over and over, I have seen effective homeopathic treatment facilitate a return to, or bring a step towards, greater wellness but most people are simply unaware of its benefits. Those that have worked with homeopathy for some time often comment that they wished they'd known about it much earlier. I am a lover of empowering people, so this book is for *you*—to share with you another option for good health that you may not know could be available to you.

Throughout our lifetimes, many of us will become 'stuck' somewhere—whether it be due to a physical, mental or emotional issue—and there are those of us that will wrestle with various health conditions for significant periods of time that perhaps could have been treated by homeopathic interventions. I know struggle can be a part of life but why should we struggle if we don't have to? As you read, I hope you can begin to see homeopathy's vast potential to assist with any number of issues in a variety of circumstances.

To start you on your own journey into homeopathy, I'll provide you with some common terms, along with their definitions. I'll also explain what homeopathy is, give a background into the field and discuss some key differences between it and conventional medicine. Next, I'll share stories of myself, family members, clients and even some beloved animals who have used homeopathy successfully. At the end of the book, you'll find some suggestions of useful books, films and websites, should you wish to explore the topic further.

While there are plenty of books, web articles, studies and more which cover extensive definitions and details of homeopathy, my aim is purely to show its potential in practical terms, using real life experiences. I've divided the stories shared here into categories, e.g. headaches and migraines, respiratory issues, mental health, etc. and will detail several of my clients' experiences in each category. In all but one instance, the cases are from my own life and clinic.

I am a huge fan of an integrative approach to wellness. I would simply like more people to be aware that homeopathy is out there so they can make an informed choice about whether or not it is for them, even if they choose not to use it. In my practice, some of my clients come fairly early to homeopathy, some have a history of taking medication for years or have had surgical or other interventions with no relief before trying homeopathy, while others have limited conventional medical options available to them from the beginning. I simply want everyone to have the best options for living life with greater ease and enjoying it to the full.

In the spirit of easing struggle and providing options, if you like the book, please share it with others. Gift it to someone you think might be helped by its contents. Shout about it to your friends. And if you try homeopathy, do share your own success stories.

I called this book *The Joy of Homeopathy* because it is a celebration—there is so much joy in what I do. There is joy in the simplicity of homeopathy; joy in finding a homeopathic medicine that matches the symptoms and the person so well that incredible things happen; joy that comes from being present, fully listening to a person as they give me a glimpse into their lives; joy in walking alongside someone through a part of their journey, whether that means helping them achieve a miraculous recovery or merely the gift of being trusted to be there during a difficult time. I hold a deep appreciation for the privilege of being with another human being and am grateful to have witnessed some extraordinary results during my time in this work.

I believe that we often have the ability to heal ourselves, and when we set up the right conditions, the process is made much easier. For me, homeopathy is a catalyst to giving our bodies what they need to get on with the healing process. I am so pleased you've decided to join me on this journey. So without further ado, let's begin!

Some Homeopathic Terminology

Before we dive in, it seems wise to explain some terminology typically used in the practice of homeopathy. If you are already familiar with these terms, feel free to skip this section; however, you may wish to return to it throughout the book to refresh your memory.

Acute
A short, time-limited illness with a clear, often rapid, onset and defined end point.

Amelioration
An improvement of symptoms. It may be a lasting improvement, which is ultimately what is desired, or temporary, which may indicate the potency or the medicine (or both) need to be changed or repeated to better match the situation.

Aggravation
A short intensification of symptoms. In the few instances when this occurs, it is usually regarded as a positive sign that the remedy is acting and is likely to be followed by an improvement of symp-

toms. However, in most cases aggravation of symptoms doesn't occur and symptoms on the whole tend to improve gently.

Chronic
From *chronos* meaning 'time'. A longer duration of illness, which may be persistent or long-lasting. Many diseases in the Western world are chronic, e.g. diabetes, autoimmune disorders, respiratory disorders or cardiovascular issues.

Dosage
The quantity and regularity of the medicine prescribed, according to the requirements of the individual and their symptoms.

First aid/minor ailment homeopathy kits
Kits produced by homeopathic pharmacies that usually contain a small number of homeopathic medicines (e.g. for two UK pharmacies this is between 18 and 42 medicines). They can be extremely useful for treating minor ailments when at home or on holiday. Some pharmacies may offer kits in different sizes and it is also possible to create your own.

Materia Medica
Latin for 'Medical Matter', *Materia Medica* books detail descriptions of homeopathic medicines and the symptoms a person may be experiencing that the medicines may help with, as discovered in provings or from clinical experience.

Medicine (see also Remedy)
Forms of treatment (e.g. a tablet or a pill, in powder form or as liquid drops in water) made to Good Manufacturing Practice (GMP) standard and regulated (in the UK) through the licensing procedures of the Medicines and Healthcare Products Regulatory Agency (MHRA).

- **Acute medicine**
  Acute medicines are selected for minor ailments and acute illnesses. In selecting a medicine for an individual, the homeopath may use symptoms relating specifically to that illness or state, without necessarily taking into account the whole person's characteristics and general ways of being.

- **Constitutional medicine**
  Constitutional medicine covers the 'bigger picture', matching the person and who they are, as well as the symptoms they're presenting with. This holistic—or whole person—approach is one of the main ways homeopathy differs from much of conventional medicine.

  (N.B. The same homeopathic medicine may be used in an acute or in a constitutional way, depending on the symptoms of the individual.)

Modalities
Modalities (or 'what makes it better or worse') are particularly helpful in homeopathic work. For example, some medicine descriptions mention symptoms that are better with rest, some with movement; some symptoms are better for heat and others for cold.

Periodic table
Created by Russian scientist Dmitri Mendeleev, who presented the table to the Russian Chemical Society in 1869. Within homeopathy, Dr Jan Scholten was a pioneer of using the periodic table in clinical practice; his observations of certain patterns within the rows and columns of the table was the start of recognising how useful it could be in homeopathy.

Polychrest
Defined as 'a thing adapted to multiple uses.'[1] In homeopathy, this

means a commonly-used medicine, often having been utilised for many years and which generally has a wide range of uses in a large number of symptoms or ailments.

Potency
The strength of a homeopathic medicine. There are three main scales of potency: the Centesimal potencies (C and M), the Decimal potencies (denoted by X) and LM potencies. Commonly prescribed potencies in homeopathy are 6X and 12X on the Decimal scale and 6C, 12C, 30C, 200C, 1M and 10M on the Centesimal scale. The LM scale starts at LM1. A fuller explanation of potencies in homeopathy is available on my website.[2] For the sake of simplicity and reader-friendliness, potencies are not detailed in the stories that follow.

Proving/prover
Provings are where participants—usually homeopathy practitioners or students—take a homeopathic medicine several times and record their responses to it. Provings are a means of discovering the effectiveness of both new as well as previously tried and tested medicines.

Remedy (see Medicine)
Whereas the medicine refers to the actual pill (or granules or drops), the remedy is the overall treatment for a particular patient or condition, which could also include changes in lifestyle and diet.

Repertory
An index of symptoms with both broad and detailed explanations. The repertory enables the homeopathic practitioner to cross-reference the symptoms of a case and assess the potential medicines in order to select the most appropriate one for that person.

Rubric

A short sentence or a few key words that describe a symptom or state. These can be more general symptoms such as 'Head, pain' (which in one repertory has 1,295 medicines listed) or more specific, individualised symptoms, e.g. 'Head pain, crossing limbs aggravates' (which has only one listed medicine).

Strange, rare or peculiar (SRP) symptoms

Strange, rare or peculiar symptoms are not seen all the time and can be symptoms that fit any (but not necessarily all) of those descriptors. These less common symptoms can be really useful in helping a homeopathic medicine be matched to the individual. Account needs to be taken of both SRP and common symptoms.[3]

Succussion

The shaking of the substance. It is thought that this is an important part in helping to 'activate' or 'energise' the medicine. Along with the dilution process, succussion has a key role in the making of homeopathic medicines.[4]

WHAT IS HOMEOPATHY?

"Homeopathy is one of the most life-changing, incredible things that I've found. I've seen it do things that nothing else can and it fascinates me all the time."

This is how I responded in a moment of clarity when I was asked to describe what homeopathy is. I really do feel this way. However, for the purpose of this book, I appreciate that I need to be a little more specific...

In short, homeopathy is a system of natural health care that has been in worldwide use in its present form for over two hundred years. This fascinates me, as many of the philosophies and much of the practice have remained unchanged, and many of the same medicines are being used for similar symptoms now as they were in the past.

The word 'homeopathy' originates from the Greek *homoios* meaning 'similar, of the same kind' and *patheia* meaning 'disease, feelings, emotions'. So the Greek word *homoiopathes* means 'having similar feelings or affections'.[1] Or, as I learnt in college, *homoeo*

= similar and *pathos* = suffering, which I feel translates a little easier into modern language. So essentially, homeopathy means 'similar suffering'. This may make a little more sense when we talk about the concept of 'like cures like' a little later.

The more I work with homeopathy and understand its overriding philosophies and principles, the more it strikes me that the concepts are, in many cases, universal (or at least well-known). Dr Christian Friedrich Samuel Hahnemann (commonly referred to as Dr Samuel Hahnemann), the founder of homeopathy, was incredibly well-read, with a diverse range of interests beyond the narrower orthodox medical view of the time. Within the tenets of homeopathy, you can find nods to many earlier philosophers and whilst Hahnemann doesn't give specific mention to Paracelcus[2] within his works, there are noticeable similarities on homeopathic thinking between Hahnemann's and the earlier Swiss-German medic's writings.[3]

Ultimately, what Hahnemann wanted to achieve, and what all of the following laws of homeopathy lead up to, is this key principle: the 'highest ideal of cure is a rapid, gentle and permanent restoration of the health, or removal and annihilation of the disease, in the shortest, most reliable and most harmless way, on easily comprehensible principles.'[4] Homeopathy aims not to suppress symptoms but to restore a patient to full health. Hahnemann in his *The Organon of Medicine* goes into detail about the principles of homeopathy, and gives clear instruction around the practice of it. Whilst I want to keep this introduction brief, I do want to mention several of the important foundations of homeopathy.

The Law of Minimum Dose: When talking about homeopathy, the philosophy of 'less is more' is crucial. This notion has recently become popular with the rise of the minimalist culture in Western societies, yet in the centuries-old practice of homeopathy, it's one of its basic concepts. The phrase 'less is more' is first found in print in 1855 in the Robert Browning poem *Andrea del Sarto*.[5] However, the idea appeared within literature much before that, particularly in the work of the aforementioned Paracelcus, to whom the quote, 'The dose makes the poison' is attributed.[6] This quote alludes to the fact that even things that are good for us can be harmful when consumed in too great a quantity—drinking enough water is sensible but drinking too much can cause catastrophic complications. The Law of Minimum Dose means a patient is only given the minimum amount of a substance needed to stimulate the patient's own healing response. My feeling is that the medicine acts almost as a catalyst, setting up conditions for the body to start healing itself. One of Hahnemann's many acts of genius was in potentising plants and other materials by succussing and diluting them in order to take substances, convert them into powerful medicines and then repeat the dose as necessary.

In Hahnemann's seminal work *The Organon of Medicine*, he counsels that only one homeopathic medicine should be prescribed at a time, rather than a combination of several medicines. This is known as **The Law of Simplex** and allows the homeopath to be able to observe the patient's response to that medicine to determine whether it fits well with the patient and their symptoms. There is some deviance from this principle at times, and it's fair to say that there are different schools of thought in the world of homeopathy on this law; however, it is my preferred way to work as well. As you'll see in most of the stories here, whilst I might give a combination remedy or more than one homeopathic medicine on occasion, I typically begin (and frequently continue) with just one.

A third homeopathic philosophy to consider is **The Law of Similars**, otherwise known as 'like cures like'. You are probably familiar with the phrase 'a little bit of what makes you ill can make you better' and I mentioned earlier that the Greek word *homoiopathes* means 'having similar feelings or affections'. Hippocrates is quoted as saying, 'A disease develops by means of its like and is cured by means of the use of its like.'[7] As with other ideologies, this concept pre-dates homeopathic philosophies and is integral to working with homeopathy.

'Like cures like' as a concept exists today in many places around us. The hangover cure 'hair of the dog' is one place we see it—the symptoms that result from too much alcohol the night before can often be relieved by an alcoholic drink the next morning. It is also seen in the conventional medical world, albeit, as with the alcohol example, without the other homeopathic principles running alongside it. Examples include the stimulant *Ritalin*, prescribed for children and adults who may experience an inability to concentrate due to over-stimulation, and in giving peanuts in minute doses to people with severe peanut allergies.[8]

A fourth philosophy, and one you'll see demonstrated throughout this book, is that of **Individualisation**. This means looking at who the person is and how they experience their unique symptoms, rather than simply assuming that a certain homeopathic medicine will work for a particular condition. Hippocrates is reported to have said, 'It is more important to know what person the dis-ease has than what dis-ease the person has.' You may notice my hyphenation of the word 'dis-ease' in this Hippocratic quote. More and more I think of it like this instead of all one. It helps me recognise the 'lack of ease', which doesn't always have to be labelled a 'disease'. The situation or symptoms may merely feel difficult, awkward or uncomfortable for the person experiencing life with less ease. Of course, I want to know the details of the symptoms that have brought you to see me but also, and super importantly, who are you? How do you experience the world?

The Dutch homeopath Dr Annette Sneevliet talks about our 'program'. Dr Rajan Sankaran, an Indian homeopath, talks about our 'non-human song'. I love both of these expressions. My job is to understand the 'song' you are singing or the 'program' or pattern that you are expressing. In terms of my own interpretation, I think of it almost as a lens that you see the world through—and this differs vastly from person to person. When we take a well-matched homeopathic medicine, it can almost feel as if we're seeing the world differently, with more clarity and more ease. This may show up as a feeling of spaciousness, an ability to observe instead of reacting immediately, a knack to viewing life with more humour, a new sense of calmness or a capacity to sleep more soundly. I often hear my clients describe a generalised sense of greater well-being along with the amelioration of their symptoms.

If I can really understand you and how you experience your dis-ease and the world around you on a more holistic level, then I'm much more likely to see a good—even great—result in clinic. I would say that's where I see my best work. One client returned to me a month after our initial session and told me with surprise, 'People smile!' She'd been so stressed—living in pain and busy doing the daily grind—that she didn't smile at others or notice they might be doing so to her. It was only when her symptoms were somewhat relieved that she was able to see the smiles of others and to smile more herself and was completely amazed that people smiled back at her. It was as if her lens on the world had become clearer and she was able to notice herself and those around her in a more compassionate way.

A fifth concept is **Holism or Totality**, where we look at the *whole person*, not just the part that has the symptoms. It might seem strange—within our modern medical paradigm—to think that a physical symptom could have anything to do with an emotional one (such as grief, for example) but I've seen it many times in practice. The whole certainly *is* greater than the sum of its parts and, in my clinic, I've seen that philosophy demonstrated over and over again.

Another important law or guideline to consider is Dr Constantine Hering's **Law of Cure**. Like Hahnemann, Hering came about this law from clinical experience. The Law of Cure states that healing happens from above downwards, from inside to outwards, from the more central to the more peripheral, from more important organs to less important ones and in the reverse order of disease appearance. These paths of healing are commonly observed phenomena within homeopathic practice and are frequently an indication that we're on the right track with our clients. For example, skin symptoms that were suppressed years ago may pop up again as a deeper issue heals. This would demonstrate three of Hering's Law of Cure observations: 1) from inside outwards, 2) more important organs to less important ones (whilst the skin is amazing, an infection or irritation on the skin is usually less serious than one in, say, the heart or brain) and 3) in reverse order of disease appearance. Often the same homeopathic medicine, if it fits the person well, may help clear new conditions as well as old, though in some cases, more than one medicine may be used.

So to sum up, what is homeopathy? As you've learned about the overriding philosophy and the laws that govern the practice, I hope it's clear that it is an approach to health and wellness that treats each person as a unique individual, with the aim of stimulating the body's own healing ability. As you'll read repeatedly throughout this book, this aspect of individuality is crucial; while working with someone, a homeopath's aim is to select the most appropriate medicine based on the individual's specific symptoms and personal level of overall health. As we head into a discussion on some of the key differences between conventional medicine and homeopathy, I want to say that, whilst this individualised approach is something that I believe is missing at times in conventional medicine, I'm seeing a real shift in that world too, with an increasing focus on the individual. This is a theme that runs through our work, and you'll hopefully see it demonstrated throughout the story section of this book, time and again.

HOMEOPATHY AND CONVENTIONAL MEDICINE

I love seeing how homeopathy or other complementary and alternative medicines (CAM) can sit alongside more conventional medical approaches. It's not a solo crusade for me—I enjoy working with people who have a team, which may include: a General Practitioner (GP), secondary medical services, a naturopath, a nutritionist, a dentist, a physiotherapist, a massage therapist, an osteopath, a functional medicine practitioner, an acupuncturist or any other therapeutic approach in between. I'm not in any way suggesting we need all of these interventions at the same time—using too many (or flitting between) approaches can be a challenge when trying to understand what is actually helping—but also, please don't go it alone!

My dream is for the worlds of CAM and conventional medicine to work together, hand-in-hand. This feels a very exciting place to me as we each have amazing things to offer in our own ways. Emergency services, surgical interventions and conventional medicines are all potentially life-saving and can bring about amazing results. In addition, conventional systems are often able to identify issues (their diagnostics are exemplary) and I frequently encourage clients to go for tests and investigations as I have neither the equipment nor the training to diagnose, and that's not my role. Still, there can often be homeopathic medicines that may support conventional interventions. For example, do not come to me with a broken leg, at least not until it's been set and dealt with at an appropriate hospital or clinic. You might come to me, however, for medicine to help the bone set quicker. I've lost count of the number of times clients have told me their doctor was amazed at how fast they healed when supported by homeopathic medicines.

But what if you have a diagnosis, particularly of the chronic kind, and there are no suitable options offered which can help restore you to good health? No one system can do everything and none of us have all the answers. Collaboration and communication with respect for the wisdom and talents of each other would seem to be of value, especially to the most important person in the room—the patient. Imagine a world where fewer hospital admissions were needed and where people could be empowered to improve their health themselves, working with a range of practitioners using gentle, effective medicines. This is my dream and I think it is achievable.

Before we take a look at some real life homeopathy stories, let's further this discussion by taking a look at how homeopathy typically differs from conventional medicine.

SOME KEY DIFFERENCES BETWEEN HOMEOPATHY AND CONVENTIONAL MEDICINE

1. The 'one size fits all' approach vs individualisation

In general, when visiting the GP, a patient with eczema will likely receive a topical treatment to apply to the skin, a complaint around a headache may result in painkillers being prescribed and depression may be treated with anti-depressants. It's not that there's anything wrong with this approach, and it can certainly be effective, but it's focused on *the part that is suffering* rather than *the person who is suffering.* This is the opposite of Hippocrates' pronouncement that it's more important we know the person who has the dis-ease than the dis-ease that has the person.

In working with homeopathy, we aim to individualise. For instance, in the repertory program I use, I have 1,295 different medicines that 'experience' headaches, so homeopaths like myself must find out more about the specific symptoms. What do the headaches feel like? What brings them on? Where do you feel them in your head? Is there any other symptom that occurs alongside them? What makes them better? What makes them worse? Do you crave any different foods or drinks at the time of your headaches? Was there anything significant happening around the time they started? In my own experience, I find that learning about the person is often a helpful key to the case, and I'll be sharing more about that as you read onwards.

When we are in pain or struggling with a symptom, we may look for that one thing—the holy grail—to 'fix' us but in the world of homeopathy, it would be folly to suggest that there's only *one* medicine out there for each individual. As we go through different situations, phases and ailments and our bodies change with time and circumstances, we can understand that we are all individuals who respond differently to the world around us. It makes sense that if we each have our own subconscious program giving us a unique lens with which we view the world, we may require a different medicine than someone else with a similar condition. And as homeopathy works with the whole person, it is easy to see why it's fairly common for someone taking a well-matched homeopathic medicine to shift their perspective along with their symptoms, allowing them to take the world (and themselves) better in stride, which may help support them to create a more fulfilling life. It's not just about the symptoms; in fact, the opposite tends to be true.

Another benefit to seeing a client as both whole and unique is that it can help prevent potential misunderstandings. For example, I may see purple but you may well see blue. Rather than presume we both see the same colour, I'm going to ask questions so as not to make an assumption that may or may not be accurate.

What I'm describing here is a holistic approach that is in contrast to the more reductionist way in which Western (conventional) medicine often tends to operate. Generally, if we visit our GP with a condition, we are not usually questioned about our lifestyle, diet, rest or exercise regime, sleeping pattern and so on. Admittedly, this may often be due to a time limitation (which I discuss below), however, as mentioned at the end of the last chapter, I'm grateful to be seeing a shift towards more lifestyle-oriented approaches. Things like social prescribing (a practice of referring patients to local, non-clinical services that can help support a person's health journey) are gaining popularity, as is a 'bigger picture' look at what constitutes 'health care'. Practitioners such as Dr Rangan Chatterjee[1] have brought lifestyle medicine to the fore and organisations like Nutritank,[2] who are passionately pioneering nutritional and lifestyle approaches in medical training, have much to be thanked for this also.

2. The unprejudiced observer

In homeopathy, we put a lot of focus during training and in practice on working towards being 'the unprejudiced observer'. To use a simple example, if we were to see a client who looks like someone else who did well on a certain homeopathic medicine or who has the same medical condition, we could make the assumption that that's what we need to give this person too. But this would be acting from a place of prejudice. This new client's internal experience of the world may be vastly different from the previous client's, despite a similar external appearance or same disease label. Whilst it is perhaps a high goal (it's almost impossible for humans to be completely objective), the more we as practitioners can work towards an unbiased view of each person, the better we'll be at our role.

*3. In addition to symptoms, homeopathic textbooks describe people,
   characteristics and conditions*

The more cases we see where a particular remedy is helpful, the
more we can build up an awareness of a medicine's potential. Creating a 'remedy picture'—an understanding of what can be helped
with each homeopathic medicine and what type of people they
work well with—is very useful. Rather than just the physical symptoms that can be helped with a specific medicine, homeopathic
resources tell us about personality types, mental and emotional
states, characteristics, dreams, fears, desires and so much more.
I've heard of more than one medical student and practitioner say
how amazed they were by the depth of descriptions in the *Materia
Medica* and other sources, leading them to want to study homeopathy as a result of reading the rich information contained within
them.

To that end, I like to tell clients (particularly children) that there
is no right or wrong in my room. In the outside world, we often
judge aspects of ourselves as either good or bad but this can, at
times, exacerbate a problem. While I'm not advocating a society
without morals or certain behaviours, if a person only presents
their 'good side' in my clinic space, it makes my work far more
challenging. I want to understand you—*all of you*—so please bring
in whatever anxieties you might hide in the outside world. I offer
you a safe space to share them.

As a reminder, the intention of this book is to provide an insight
into the potential of homeopathy, rather than a detailed textbook
on the subject. As a result, the descriptions of the people highlighted in the cases, and the particular medicines used, are purposefully
kept brief. There is already so much written about homeopathy—there are so many wonderful texts out there, including many
brilliant *Materia Medica* resources—that instead, I want you to
experience how the medicines work through the stories of those
who were helped by them. However, if you're intrigued and want

to find out more, please go out and explore! Do also check out the resources located at the back of this book.

4. *Length of consultation*

In a system that customarily permits us a mere ten minutes to discuss our most pressing health concerns with our GP, my allocation of between one-and-a-half and two hours for an initial consultation with a client could seem like an eternity. Not all homeopathic practitioners offer sessions of that duration but I personally tend to operate within this time allotment. My follow-up sessions are generally thirty to sixty minutes long.

However we work as homeopaths, you will likely find us scheduling longer sessions than you are probably used to. This gives us time to explore those two critical aspects: who you are and how you experience your symptoms. A typical consultation is not a 'quick fire of symptoms then away with a suggestion of a homeopathic medicine' kind of scenario. A homeopath asks questions, allows time for you to talk and has developed excellent listening skills. And while we get the answers we need in order to suggest a matching remedy, there is often a benefit from simply being heard too; clients have told me they understand their issues much better after having discussed them, enabling them to make connections on their own that they hadn't been able to before.

I was several years into practice when I recognised that it would be incredibly arrogant of me to think I can understand the whole of a person after just two hours. Like most trained practitioners—conventional, homeopathic or otherwise—I'm always eager for everyone to feel better yesterday but at times, it can be more of a process than a quick fix. Healing often isn't linear—it can be more like peeling the layers of an onion. In those cases where I don't seem to get right to the heart of the matter straight away, this analogy can be really helpful to remember. Often, as a client gets comfortable working with me, more information comes to light, illuminating another aspect that is meant to be helped.

5. Recognising the psychological roots of illness

Sometimes we have an inkling of where something 'came from'. Years ago, I experienced post-traumatic stress disorder-like symptoms following a house fire two doors down from us. I was awoken at two a.m. by a neighbour hammering on our front door yelling, 'The house is on fire!' As if that wasn't bad enough, the house in flames had an ammunition cupboard in the loft. To add to my experience, I'd been reading a novel which featured Hutu and Tutsi conflicts and had just finished a section in which a hospital had been broken into and people were sheltering in cupboards trying to avoid being gunned down. Waking to the sound of banging on the door, shots apparently being fired and people yelling and screaming, I managed to convince myself that someone outside was out to kill me and my young daughter. Thus began a heightened state of anxiety and an adrenaline-like feeling that lasted for quite some time after the event.

This is a clear example of what is termed an 'exciting cause'—an event, experience or shock that may trigger a health issue. It was weeks before the 'running on adrenaline' feeling dissipated and I could sleep soundly through the night. Although I was confident that I could take homeopathic medicines to ease the condition, I decided not to as I wanted to gain a greater awareness of what others may be going through when they talk about traumatic situations in their own lives. Of course, I appreciate that someone else encountering the exact same thing would likely experience it very differently, but going through this ordeal gave me a flavour of dealing with the aftermath of a trauma-inducing event. I'm not sure I'd stoically carry on now—I was younger then and nowadays I'd probably dive into the homeopathy cupboard earlier—but I'm still grateful to have experienced that state for my own understanding.

In clinic, I sometimes see physical symptoms that stem from emotions such as grief, heartbreak, excitement, worry or fear. No one has told me yet that they got overly joyful and then their arthritis started (though never say never!). It's generally the 'negative' experiences that cause physical ailments, especially if we've suppressed our emotions in the name of 'getting on with it'. So many of us are good at keeping things in check and being 'fine' but I'm not sure it's always fine for our bodies. Even with the best will in the world, events in our lives can still have an impact on us and coping with events in the aftermath can absolutely be part of what we need to help within our homeopathic practice rooms. Whether you seek out homeopathy or not, fully processing events with a therapist, a journal or a friend is surely healthier than keeping it all inside.

6. Everything is useful

Medical homeopath Dr Julie Geraghty,[3] previously a General Practitioner, says that patients used to tell her things that she had 'no way of making sense of' as a conventional doctor. It wasn't even so much that she didn't have the time to talk to the patient (although there could be that, too), it was that she had no frame of reference for how to apply some of the details that were given.

Once she started practising homeopathy, she realised she could often use more of the information she gained in session to get to the roots of the illness and, therefore, be in a better position to help her patients restore their health. The times people wake and sleep, what they desire to eat and drink, their dreams, fears and anxieties can all—along with their symptoms—give us insights into selecting particular homeopathic medicines to suit that person, but that just wasn't part of a GP's training.

7. The placebo effect

The placebo effect (placebo is Latin for 'I shall please') is described as 'a beneficial effect in a patient following a particular treatment that arises from the patient's expectations concerning the treatment rather than from the treatment itself.'[4] At times the term can be used in a dismissive way, as an explanation for the efficacy of homeopathic treatment.

Placebo as a concept definitely fascinates me. It seems that across the board, in whatever healing paradigm, we see a percentage of people get better as the sole result of their thoughts and beliefs about the treatment they receive. Figures vary, but in one study nearly half the people who underwent simulated surgery as part of a clinical trial were feeling better six months after the procedure.[5] In a review of studies on antidepressants and the placebo effect, between thirty and forty percent of participants got relief despite not taking the active drug.[6] There is something quite incredible going on here. The idea that humans may feel better by simply verbalising their distress in an atmosphere of non-judgment and kindness, or when receiving a diagnosis and being given something that is deemed a remedy (even if it's a sugar pill), makes sense. But how does that work in animals?

Our horse (to our awareness) probably thought she was eating a tasty chunk of carrot. It's unlikely she noticed the medicine hidden in it. I've heard passionate advocates of the placebo effect expound that the animal sensed the owner was feeling calmer, which allowed for the animal to improve. Perhaps—taken on face value—they may have a point but most animals treated with homeopathy first went down a route of conventional medicine that hadn't helped them. Surely homeopathic vets aren't *that* much more sympathetic and kinder than conventional vets? The theory doesn't hold up for me, at least in the realm of homeopathy.

It's not unusual for homeopaths to see high improvement rates in their clinics and a large scale study conducted at Bristol Homeopathic Hospital, published in 2005, saw around a seventy percent improvement rate.[7] Whilst 'it's just placebo' may be a criticism that's often flung at homeopaths, the figures from plentiful research and our experiences in clinic suggest the results are well beyond what is typically known as accounting for this effect. At times—as you'll read in the stories—I'll suggest a medicine that doesn't fully match the individual and we won't see the change that both I and the client are hoping for. I'm content to see people respond quickly to homeopathic medicines time and again when the right medicine is given.

8. Costs of treatment

There have been some in-depth studies of the costs associated with homeopathic treatment as compared to conventional medicine. The results are varied. A small study undertaken in Italy between 1998 and 2003 showed that the costs of homeopathic treatment for respiratory diseases were significantly lower than those for conventional pharmacological therapy,[8] while a larger German study published in 2017 showed higher costs in the homeopathy group compared to the control group.[9] Another study involving 493 participants, published in 2005, found similar costs between the conventional and homeopathic groups, but also that the patients using homeopathic treatment had a better outcome overall.[10] Because homeopathic treatment is highly individualised, it's certainly difficult to compare a treatment for say, a short-lasting respiratory condition with a much more complex case. There's no 'one size fits all' here, which makes studying this issue complicated.

However, the actual cost of the treatment is only one part of the equation. In the same way that the cost of organic food is typically higher than food which is far more processed (with the potential harmful side effects and environmental repercussions that entails), it can be argued that homeopathy is a much more sustainable medicine. As it is often better for both our bodies and the environment—and comes with fewer side effects—sometimes it's worth paying a little more. I would add that what I've seen in clinic supports the fact that it's generally more cost-effective too. We also need to remember that when we're using state-provided health services, we don't always perceive the real cost of treatment; the time spent with our GP can feel like it's cost-free but, of course, it's not. And while defining the cost effectiveness of homeopathy continues to be a matter for ongoing discussion, the experience of rediscovering your health through homeopathy could be considered priceless!

9. Invasive, long-term vs non-invasive, short-term treatment

In my experience, using homeopathy may help us avoid the need for surgery, as well as assist in reducing or eliminating medication. You'll read in the pages to come that in some cases, invasive treatment was avoided for some of the individuals concerned.

One client, who had been advised he would need surgery for tendonitis in his shoulder, demonstrated to me how he couldn't raise his arm above his head. After giving him a homeopathic medicine, he returned to see me about four weeks later, showed me the full raising of his arm and told me it was fine now after the remedy, without surgical intervention. My partner Steve—whose story features in the Skin Complaints section—avoided having minor surgery to deal with a cyst on his scalp after taking several homeopathic medications. Kay—in the Respiratory Issues section—had already had two surgical interventions but was still left dealing with copious amounts of mucus on a daily basis. After six homeopathic consultations, and several repetitions of the same homeopathic medicine, she described how she was ninety-nine percent better, which leads me to wonder if it would have been possible to avoid those surgeries altogether? And you've already heard that Kara, our horse, avoided surgery to remove her eye. Years later I happened to meet Chris Day and his wife, who told me that they'd seen horses have an eye removed as treatment for uveitis, only to have the other eye affected by it too.

My client Sarah had been taking anti-depressants for many years and was able to reduce the dose, then come off them altogether, by using homeopathy and reducing her anti-depressant medications in consultation with her doctor. Laura had 'tried nearly everything' to help her dermatitis; after using homeopathy, it fully resolved for her. Afterwards, she described her experience with homeopathy as 'magic'.

I don't think of homeopathy as an either/or to conventional medicine and, hopefully, you'll feel the same way after reading this book. I wouldn't want to live in a world where surgery and conventional medications aren't offered or available; they are frequently brilliant and can certainly be life-saving. I believe there's a place for us all. That said, working with homeopathy alongside can help us cope with the side effects of conventional medications, ease post-surgical recovery and at times, reduce the need for them altogether. In my experience as a client and practitioner, I've seen that homeopathy can help restore health, in the words of Hahnemann, 'gently, permanently and rapidly' without us needing other interventions.

10. Sustainable/eco-friendly medicine

Because of the very nature of homeopathic medicine, no toxic side products are created in their manufacturing, and original substances are sustainably sourced. In addition, we only need a small amount of something to be able to create a homeopathic medicine, and many pills in various potencies can be medicated from this. This potentially makes homeopathy one of the most eco-friendly forms of medicine out there!

11. Side effects

Some people say that homeopathy has no side effects. I feel like I can't fully agree with this as there are times when we can see an aggravation or intensification of symptoms. The good news is, this is fairly rare and is frequently a sign that the homeopathic medicine chosen is a good match. It's almost like the symptoms are pushed a little further before coming back to a place of equilibrium.

With homeopathy, if an aggravation should occur, it is generally short-lasting and can be dealt with quickly. Interestingly, the side effects of some conventional medicines are one of the reasons many people are drawn to homeopathy in the first place. For example, in pregnancy or with young children, conventional medication may carry risks that have to be weighed against the benefits and this is an area where homeopathy comes into its own. It has a very low risk of side effects and is safe to use for all ages.

As you'll read in the stories section, the risk of taking a medication for her ulcerative colitis symptoms whilst breastfeeding didn't appeal to Maayan, and she was able to manage her symptoms successfully using homeopathy instead. Similarly, you'll read about Louise, who was coping with side effects of other treatments and was offered a drug that had the risk of 'putting her into a vegetative state'. Her symptoms had become so intense that she was considering it, but fortunately, homeopathy helped to make things much more manageable for her without going down that road.

12. Empowering self-care

To be able to do something to help yourself without needing to call on others is a major bonus, and one that is so rarely an option in our current health care environment. Of course, we need to refer to medical help where needed and we don't want to mess around in an emergency. Still, I've heard of more than a few stories of someone in acute pain calling for medical help, popping a homeopathic medicine while they waited and being fine by the time they arrived at a hospital or saw a doctor. I always recommend setting the wheels in motion, then taking to the books or the kit. It's amazing what these small pills can do—but don't delay seeking medical assistance.

Getting started with homeopathy for minor ailments is really straightforward. A great place to begin is with a first aid kit of homeopathic medicines. The kits I mention throughout the book (available from homeopathic pharmacies—more information in the Useful Resources section) contain medicines that may help cuts heal quicker, alleviate or reduce muscle or nerve pain, heal bruising and lots more. They come with simple, easy-to-follow booklets and you can get started straight away by following the instructions. With just one homeopathic medicine—for example, Arnica—there's loads you can help yourself and your family with. It's effective in treating bruising, shocks, jet lag, tiredness (you know that feeling when you've 'hit a wall' and can't do anymore?) and that's just for starters. A client recently told me that her kit has become her most used and treasured possession and wonders how she managed for so long without one. I often suggest that people have one in their home, workplace or car. Or all three!

In addition, you can find individuals, colleges, organisations or charities that offer introductory homeopathy courses which can assist you in gaining more confidence in using these medicines for yourself and your family. There are home-study courses available at all levels as well as attendance courses. It's truly amazing what you can do for yourself and your loved ones for simple conditions with a few great medicines and some basic knowledge.

13. Instant symptom suppression vs restoring health

In homeopathy, our overall goal is for you to no longer experience the symptoms, rather than medicate to suppress them indefinitely, and I think this is often a key difference between conventional and homeopathic treatment. You're unlikely to be taking homeopathic medicines on a daily basis, let alone for life. As homeopaths, we are always aiming for the minimum dose and minimum repetition that creates a resolution of symptoms.

Going back to our horse, the homeopathic treatment involved five days of tablets. Compare this to the six-weekly steroid injections and anti-inflammatory meds that we'd been using prior to finding homeopathy. After the homeopathic remedy, she never suffered from the condition again.

In my own case, when I visited the doctors at age seventeen (as you'll read about in the stories section), I was given beta blockers to reduce my migraine headaches. This would keep them mostly at bay but wouldn't actually resolve the issue as they would come back once I stopped taking the medication. Likewise, Ann and

Karen (also featured in the Headaches and Migraines section), both took medication for years and, like me, the pills would help while they had the pain but didn't stop the headaches from returning. Yet within five months of us working together, Karen was no longer experiencing headaches and within eleven weeks, the frequency and intensity of Ann's headaches had been significantly reduced and she was using much less conventional medication. My own recovery wasn't quite that fast.

People sometimes talk about homeopaths being the hardest patients for whom to find a matching homeopathic medicine, and it definitely has been a process rather than a quick fix for me. While mine wasn't a 'sorted in five months' case, my migraines have vastly improved in frequency, intensity and duration and I've learnt and grown so much along the way.

We are all unique and healing isn't always neatly linear. Sometimes we need to change the dose or frequency of a medicine. Sometimes the medicine is a mismatch and nothing changes until we get more insight into a new way to go. Some of us are starting from a place of worse health than others (often for reasons beyond our control) and may need more time or more frequent repetition of a homeopathic medicine.

There is a simple rule of thumb in homeopathic conversation: however many years something has been an issue, that may be the amount of time in months it will take to resolve it. You've had headaches for five years? Expect to have a lot fewer of them in around five months. It's not perfect, but it does give patients an idea of the possible duration of the treatment. I've seen people take less time to get well than this rule of thumb and others take longer. We may have spent a lifetime getting to where we are now, so to turn things around instantly, although it would be nice, isn't always that realistic. That said, frequently things can resolve far quicker than we might expect. As a homeopath, I'm happy to support someone on their health journey until there is no longer a need.

'Healing' means 'restoration to health and wholeness'.[11] Homeopathic medicines are typically repeated at intervals for a period of time, as opposed to the 'take it daily' (and sometimes forever) approach. For me, the concepts of 'less is more' and 'resolve not suppress' are core differences between our homeopathic and conventional worlds. I think most people would prefer not to take medication for a lifetime. Ideally, for many of us, all we really want is to actually *be well.*

Despite everything I've just shared in this section about the effectiveness of homeopathy, there exists in the world a surprising amount of antipathy towards the practice. We'll conclude this chapter by briefly examining where this hostility may stem from and why I believe it's unfounded.

HOSTILITY TOWARDS HOMEOPATHY

Because I experience, on a daily basis, the wonders that homeopathy can achieve, I could get angry when people claim it doesn't work, that it's 'pseudoscience'. How does that help individuals who may have suffered from health challenges for years before discovering this approach to health care?

Wikipedia is a perfect example. Their page on homeopathy is 'protected' from editing by certain users and has a very anti-homeopathy slant. Several homeopathic organisations have come together to caution people to view the Wikipedia entry on homeopathy as inaccurate, heavily biased and not a credible source of information.[12] The page does not present the data objectively and factually in order to allow people to make their own informed choices. Unfortunately, any discussions about this with the founder of Wikipedia have been to no avail: the Wiki mind is made up.

The Wiki experience is nothing new; homeopathy has been suppressed for years. I recognise that homeopathy's founder, Dr Samuel Hahnemann, whilst brilliant (and in my opinion, a genius) was not massively humble. I'm fairly sure he was one of the first to start the finger-pointing; in his *The Organon of Medicine*—an incredible work—Hahnemann doesn't hold back on his contempt of the medical practices of the time.[13] Sadly, there have been two sides shouting at each other across the divide for generations.

However, one thing that amuses me in the midst of the shouting are those people who go out to 'prove' homeopathy doesn't work, that it *can't* work... then find it does. One example is Dr Constantine Hering, who was tasked with disproving homeopathy and instead of doing so, became fascinated by it. First, he repeated some of the early experiments that Hahnemann had carried out and became ever more convinced that there was something to this curious medicine. Then in 1824, after a cut finger became gangrenous and routine orthodox medicine had no effect, Hering was treated by Dr Ernst Kummer, a homeopath and disciple of Hahnemann's. Hering's finger healed and his book, meant to reveal the results of his experiments, was never published.[14] Hering went on to become known as the 'Father of American Homeopathy' and developed, among other things, the Law of Cure.[15]

As Hahnemann points out in his *Materia Medica Pura*, homeopathy is best encountered as an experiential medicine.[16] When you see it, you see it. Theoretically, we may struggle to explain it, to understand the how, and yet plenty of things present this same challenge. I know of many people who became homeopaths because they either saw how someone responded to the medicine or they themselves had an experience that changed their lives. In any case, once you've seen the beauty and potential of homeopathy, it's extremely difficult to un-see it.

That's not to say that homeopathy is not based on solid evidence, or that there aren't studies to confirm its validity. There is plenty of good evidence for those prepared to look, even when others try to debunk it. For example, Professor Robert Hahn, a leading Swedish medical researcher, wrote in a 2013 paper on meta-analyses of pooled clinical data that in order to 'conclude that homeopathy lacks clinical effect, more than 90% of the available clinical trials had to be disregarded. Alternatively, flawed statistical methods had to be applied.'[17] And Dr Peter Fisher, who was homeopath to Queen Elizabeth II until his death in 2018, was a world renowned researcher who brought much clarity to this area through his passionate and rigorous work.[18]

If you're more of a visual seeker of information than a reader of scientific papers, you might want to check out the 2017 films *Magic Pills* by Ananda More and Laurel Chiten's *Just One Drop*, or the 2024 documentary *Introducing Homeopathy* (see the Useful Resources section at the end of the book for details).

There is much to explore in this area, and I'm grateful that many passionate researchers are working on it, despite the opposition and hostility they regularly face. I am hopeful that one day, the two opposing schools of thought will be able to appreciate—or at the very least acknowledge—each other's views and contributions and work together harmoniously for the benefit of the health of each and every one of us.

REAL LIFE STORIES

'The proof is in the pudding' is a phrase I often use when I talk to clients. I like to explain why I've chosen a particular homeopathic medicine and I may feel confident I've chosen a good match, but we need to wait and see what it does—hence, 'the proof is in the pudding.' If it does nothing then I'm back to the books. However, when the remedy *does* fit well, you know it's working because you see and feel the changes. You'll read about what that might look and feel like on a personal level in the stories shared in this section.

You could also use this saying in a broader sense regarding home-opathy. As I mentioned in the last section, the scientific community and mainstream media have not always been kind to the practice of homeopathy. Still, my direct experience—and that of many of my clients, other practitioners, researchers and users of homeopathy worldwide—suggest that it has a solid place in our health and wellness toolbox. Here too, the proof is in the pudding. See what you think as you read onwards.

It's often easiest, and most enjoyable, for us to learn something new through story. It is in this spirit that I want to share the experiences of some of the people I've worked with in my practice. The following anecdotes are divided into categories that generally describe what the person initially sought help for, however, you'll also see crossovers in many of the cases. For example, you'll find Claire's case in the respiratory section as she wanted help with asthma but was also seeking help to cope with work-related stress. Maayan wanted help with headaches along with digestive symptoms and her emotional health. We are complex beings, which means that often in clinic, practitioners see lots of symptoms presented at once affecting more than one aspect of a person's life. How it all fits together is a fascinating and valuable facet of our work.

It's helpful to know, as you read these cases, that homeopaths consider symptoms as an expression of dis-ease, not the dis-ease itself. Because we are treating the individual, not a condition or label, when I meet with someone I always want to know two things: 1) the symptoms or challenges that have brought them to my clinic and 2) who they are. The 'who they are' can be quite a lot of what we cover in the consultation space and you'll get glimpses into that as you read on. We might look at likes, dislikes, emotions, where someone may feel most comfortable (e.g. their climate or location), work, hobbies, fears, dreams and lots more.

For instance, we may have had a shock or grief, as in the case of Juliet, that then may trigger a physical response, such as her skin symptoms. Understanding those symptoms in relation to what was going on in her life helped me to find a remedy that saw her skin improve as well as her feeling better mentally and emotionally. In most of the stories here, I'll be talking about what homeopaths call 'constitutional prescribing', which essentially means giving a medicine that matches the person as well as the complaint that has brought them to see me. When we treat an ailment in this way, we have a greater ability to see people move to a place of better holistic health.

As I mentioned above, I'm aware that I may feel confident I've found the best matching homeopathic medicine (it can sound great on paper!) but the remedy may not match as fully as it could and we have to go back to the drawing board. You will see, in some of these cases, just how important a follow-up appointment can be. Subsequent sessions allow us to gather more information and adjust a medicine's potency and frequency of dosage, or change the medicine itself, when needed. The cases presented in this section have been chosen as a reflection of life in clinic, not as 'perfect cases' where everything always went according to plan. Sometimes I wasn't always able to perceive the 'best remedy' immediately and, as I reiterate elsewhere in the book, sometimes it can take time.

I also want to mention that homeopathic medicines can be used by any age group. Children respond really well to them too, and because the treatments are non-toxic, easy to administer and swift-working, it's a win-win. The medicines are small, and often delivered via medicated sugar pills or in water, so there's no bad taste. Also, the medicines can work to diminish symptoms quite rapidly and like anyone, kids appreciate feeling better fast! As with any client, when well-matched with a medicine, the change can be impressive. I do think it's empowering for children to grow up learning to listen to their bodies, know what makes them better and worse and reach for something that can positively influence their own health. One young client used to go off and get the homeopathy kit and bring it back to his mum saying, 'There'll be a crunchy ball for that.' Ideally, I think working with homeopathy encourages us all to live more in tune with who we are and what we need in order to live well.

When I was a student learning homeopathy, I would often say things like, 'Oh, I do that, maybe I need that remedy?' I've heard it countless times from myself, from my classmates in my student days and now in the classroom as a lecturer. It's easy to identify with the stories of others, but I want to stress that the cases you'll be reading about are short vignettes—not the whole story.

To illustrate the diversity of conditions that may be helped with one homeopathic medicine, several of the cases feature the same medicine. For example, Lac felinum—the medicine made from cat's milk—is given in two different situations, one for a client with a skin condition and another for someone experiencing mental stress.

I also want to mention that while some clients may come to me wishing to reduce their conventional medication, it isn't my role to do that. It's very important that they look at this in consultation with the prescribing medic or medical team and I always refer people back to their doctor should they wish to do this.

I've much reduced the details and insights for clarity and ease of reading, and I want to caution you to not try constitutional prescribing at home! If you are inspired by the stories, you'll find details of where you might locate a homeopath to work with (at least for UK readers) at the back of the book, which is especially relevant if something long-standing or complex is going on.

Ideally, all of the concepts I've discussed so far will become clearer as you read your way through the stories that follow. I hope you enjoy them!

1

HEADACHES AND MIGRAINES

Headaches and migraines are commonplace in society and, having experienced significant challenges with them myself, I'm always grateful to see others find relief from them too. In 2018, it was estimated that the equivalent of 86 million workdays are lost to migraine each year in the UK, and close to £1 billion is spent on healthcare costs associated with the condition.[1] They're almost accepted as 'normal' and indeed, as you'll read, some people are told that there's nothing that can be done about them except to take painkillers. But sometimes there *is* something else that can be done. I'll start this section with my own story, then share those of Arthur, Karen and Ann of how they also used homeopathy to help with their headaches and migraines.

EM: MY OWN CASE

Migraines and headaches were the first thing that took me to see a homeopath. My experience of them started very young. I had glasses from age three, my parents realising I needed them due to my describing symptoms of frequent headaches. My migraines started in primary school—I remember having them at the age of nine or so—and they continued throughout my secondary school education. They were so debilitating I would be sent home. Once there, I'd lie in a dark room crying in pain. I would feel slightly better once I'd been sick, then would have to sleep for an hour and finally, I would be able to get up and potter about. Headache medication made some impact if taken in time, but if taken too late it did nothing.

At age seventeen, it all came to a head. I was coping with the recent death of my grandad alongside the stress of A-levels, and I ended up having a lot of migraines. Of course, the stress exacerbated them and they in turn exacerbated the stress, and I was anxious that I would be unable to revise for my exams. At the time, I was taking Paracetamol, Ibuprofen, Feverfew herbal tablets and Migraleve and didn't really know what else to do to help myself.

Visiting the GP, I was given beta blockers which, to be fair, stopped the migraines. I didn't notice any side effects of the medication (though I do recall thinking it was really cool that my resting heart rate was so low!), but I know others may have less fun with them—for some, the side effects can be pretty challenging. While the beta blockers did stop the migraines, once I stopped taking them the migraines returned. What I really wanted was a solution that was effective in resolving them permanently, or at least significantly reducing them so that I didn't have to depend on pain relief which wouldn't always work. So, since as a family we'd seen great success with our horse—and I'd run out of options that worked well for me—it meant it was now my turn to sit in the homeopath's consulting room.

In my case, using homeopathy alongside other integrative approaches was the start of a journey that would make much more sense to me than taking medications that didn't always prove effective. It would also help me understand myself in a new way. One of the insights that came from those early sessions was that I was used to taking myself fairly seriously at times. I had wanted to be a vet from age seven and, as veterinary school is extremely competitive, I knew early on I needed to succeed academically. I was happy to work hard, and school work wasn't terribly difficult for me, but it was so important to me to do well and to 'get it right'. As the pressure mounted at the selective, all-girls secondary school I attended, I would put more and more pressure upon myself. One of the questions the homeopath asked me at the time—how do you express your anger?—got my attention. I remember telling her I didn't really experience anger. At the time I thought this was a good thing, but years later, I realised that's not always a healthy position. Was it possible I tended to suppress negative emotions which, along with the pressure, was potentially contributing to my headaches? It was certainly feasible. To be fair, I had a pretty great upbringing and there wasn't a huge amount for me to get angry about. Still, learning how to *express* some emotions better, rather than repress them, has contributed to my overall well-being over time.

The first homeopathic medicine I was given was Natrum muriaticum and looking back, it makes a lot of sense to me that I was given that. I was quite reserved, polite, studious, loved being by the sea, was better in open air—and with these awful headache challenges, the remedy fitted well. It was a great place to start, and the homeopathic medicine that I've found most effective relates to it closely.

Today, I still get the occasional headache or migraine; it's a susceptible area for me. We all have different weak spots, and headaches and migraines are one of mine. That said, compared to the frequency, intensity and duration I experienced when they first began, my headaches have improved in all areas and homeopathy has been one of the most effective things I've used to help them.

Arthur

Arthur was ten when we first met. He would have migraines, often brought on by excitement. A holiday, birthday, Christmas and the like were all occasions that might trigger a migraine, though other stressors could bring them on too. My own migraines sounded like a walk in the park compared to Arthur's! He would often get into periods of cyclical vomiting and, more than once, he ended up in hospital with these episodes. My first plan of action was giving a constitutional remedy that hopefully would help by reducing the frequency and intensity of his migraines.

You might think the consultation begins when you sit down and start talking, and of course an element of it does. However, we can also pick up clues as to who a person is on the very first encounter with them. 'Who a person is' is what fascinates me most in my search for a homeopathic medicine—on a constitutional level at least. 'Who is Arthur?' 'Who is it that is having these migraines?' I can glean a lot through simple observation, even before the conversation begins. It might not change the questions I'll be asking, but it's an insight into who I'm meeting.

Arthur strode into my house and walked with a not cocky, but very self-assured air... in the wrong direction. 'We're up there,' I commented. 'Ah, okay,' he replied without missing a beat. I noticed that he didn't wait to be told what to do and the way he carried himself and interacted with me on a variety of topics was with more confidence than I would have expected for a child of his age. As an observation by itself, that could lead to many places, but there are certain homeopathic medicine pictures that describe someone who is naturally more or less confident. For me, the fact that he was in a new situation, displaying an amount of composure beyond his years and not typical of his peers, was important to note.

A likeable boy, he was fascinated by outer space. I had no idea, for some of the session, what we were really talking about—black holes eating matter, exploding elements to create new unheard of elements and lots more. He described how he and his friend were the only two in his class who 'had a few brain cells' and how the other boys spent their breaks playing football. The autonomy he displayed—being willing to follow his own path—and the trust he had in himself, amongst other aspects, led me to select the homeopathic medicine Gadolinium in a high potency.

After taking the remedy, Arthur's migraines hugely reduced, both in intensity and frequency, quite quickly. When they did occur, they were usually much shorter and less severe than they'd previously been and with far fewer of the vomiting episodes. The family could finally go on holiday without fear of one of them coming on. One Christmas, however, he was back to having the cyclical vomiting experience. His mum had a homeopathic first aid kit at home and she gave him a few medicines, as well as some others I'd suggested but nothing was helping. She'd also called the National Health Service helpline, who said if he didn't improve shortly she should bring him into Accident and Emergency (A&E).

So, back to the books. We looked again at his symptoms and I took into account particularly those that were acute. Looking again in detail at the nausea, trembling and vomiting during the headaches, as well as the fact they tended to occur after emotional excitement, I decided to give the homeopathic medicine Aethusa as an acute treatment for his current state. Aethusa is a medicine I hadn't used before (and to date not used

Aethusa

since), but it has characteristic symptoms relating to the brain and nervous system (Arthur's migraines) connected with gastrointesti-

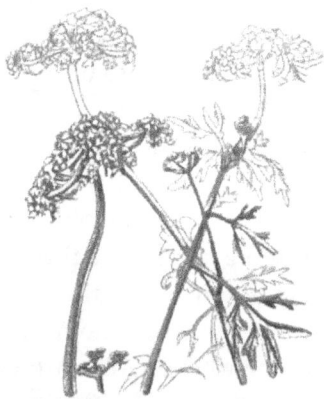

nal disturbance (his vomiting) and felt like a good match for what he was experiencing.

Since we were due to travel past Arthur's house on our way to visit friends, in the spirit of the holiday (it was Christmas after all) we dropped the medicine off. Within ten minutes of us having made the delivery, I got a text message from his mum to let me know that he was now out of bed—the first time in a few days—and was downstairs chatting to friends. She wrote, 'I can't believe it. He's like a different child to half an hour ago!' She reported that he was able to eat and drink that afternoon and was so much better. Arthur continued to improve and the next day, when his symptoms got a little worse again, the remedy was repeated, leading to a full recovery. Best of all, he didn't have to be admitted to hospital at Christmas. His mum told me that Arthur made a toast at their Christmas Eve dinner that night: 'To Em Colley, who saved Christmas!'

This case remains with me as a testimony to the potential for a vast and speedy improvement when you get *that medicine* which matches the symptoms beautifully.

KAREN

Karen and I first met in 2013, when she was fifty-nine. A mutual friend suggested she come to see me, but it was with reluctance that she did so. Karen had been advised by her GP years ago that there was nothing she could do for her headaches but keep taking the painkillers. She took Paracetamol, as and when needed, and got on with living with the headaches as best as she could. She would often take up to four lots of Paracetamol in a day—some days it might be just two tablets but more likely it was six or eight. At one point she had suffered with full blown migraines, which acupuncture had helped to resolve, but the headaches themselves remained. And because the pain never seemed to go away completely—sometimes 'hovering' for up to ten days at a time—Karen felt as if she was living with a permanent headache. Working together, we discovered there absolutely *was* something she could do. Let me tell you a little more.

Karen worked both a full-time, forty-hour-a-week job (which was fairly stressful) and a part-time job for a family business at the weekend. In addition, her elderly mother needed a lot of support from her. Karen's lack of self-confidence was also an issue. She said, 'If I was to describe myself I'd say, "I'm nothing. I never do my best in others' eyes."' She told me she was permanently in her head, saying things like, 'I'm not good enough. How can I be good enough?' Though she appeared outwardly confident, it would take her a tremendous amount of effort just to walk through the door of a Pilates class because she was constantly fighting with these thoughts about herself and what others perceived of her, causing her to retreat inwards and withdraw from everything. Karen also told me about her sixth sense—for example, she would always know when her mother was about to call—but growing up, she had been called 'fanciful' and told she was 'away with the fairies.' The combination of all of this had her feeling as if nothing in her life was working.

Many homeopathic medicines will have headaches in the rubrics (the list of symptoms) because it's such a common human experience. Taking into account Karen's low self-esteem, her concern about what others thought of her, her intuitive side and her feelings of embarrassment and guilt, I checked to see what homeopathic medicine might help her. Looking back at the work I did on Karen's case, I didn't end up choosing any rubrics that actually mentioned headaches, however, I did check the *Materia Medica* to ensure they could be relevant to the medicine I selected.

I chose a medicine called Kali bromatum in a high potency and asked her to take just two doses. This medicine has been around for a long time in homeopathy, dating back to 1838. It has a wide range of uses, but it's not one that I've given anyone with headaches before or since. However, Kali brom seemed to fit key aspects of who Karen was as part of the bigger picture. Her extreme lack of self-confidence and outlook on life (which had a lot to do with work, duty, tasks, doing the right thing and feelings of guilt) all matched the medicine well.

When we met a month later, she described feeling 'a bit lighter, more upright' within the first few days of taking it, and her headaches had reduced in severity from ten out of ten to five out of ten. I often ask clients to rate how things are in percentages or on a scale of one to ten as it makes it clearer for me—and for them—how much things have improved and where they haven't. Excitingly, Karen also told me that there were incidents that had occurred over the last month which in the past would have stressed her out, but now she was more able to let them go. 'Something else has happened too,' she told me. 'Before, I would want to make excuses all the time, but now I can stop myself. I used to text lengthy explanations to someone in order to explain. Now I just state the facts.' She also recounted an incident that normally would have made her turn away and cry but this time she spoke up, recognising she wasn't in the wrong. I asked about her need to withdraw and she told me she no longer wanted to do that. She added, 'Before, I was letting the world batter me around the head. I don't think it's my lot anymore.'

It's likely not a coincidence that she used the words 'batter me around the head.' It's amazing how often someone may say something like, 'it's eating me up inside' when they've come to talk to me about their irritable bowel or 'it's doing my head in' when describing their migraines. Our language can echo a deep and unconsciousness awareness of ourselves that is truly awe-inspiring, and our job as homeopaths is to listen well because these subtleties are often very relevant.

Meeting again a month later, Karen said her headaches had improved a little. She was still taking Paracetamol, though not as many as before. On average now, if she got a headache she only ever took one tablet and that would be enough for it to go. She mentioned in the past how she used to panic if she couldn't find her tablets and how that feeling had improved. She also said, 'I seem to have a bit more space in my head. The headaches seemed to take up a lot of space but, now they've reduced, I have more room for remembering things.' She went on to say, 'It's exhausting having headaches all the time. Not having them constantly has lightened up things that used to be a chore. Since the homeopathy, I've not had endless time with a headache and that's amazing for me.' Karen further explained, 'I think before, I was just existing, just getting through every month that went by. Now, I tell myself that this moment in time will never happen again, so I let it go. I can't believe I lived like that. I did do things and I laughed but there was always the headaches and fear of the headaches at the back of my mind. The fact I've not got a pain in my head [right now] is amazing.' More and more, she felt she was taking things easier and letting go so there was also less fight. She told me, 'I think I've been my biggest problem.' My feeling as a practitioner is that a well-matching homeopathic medicine often helps us to see ourselves and the world around us with more clarity.

We had monthly follow-ups and at our session five months after our initial meeting, Karen's headache update felt particularly significant. When I asked her about her headaches, she told me, 'I don't seem to even get them anymore. I was lying in bed yesterday and I couldn't remember when I last had one.' I was delighted for her and she was even more so! We've continued to work together since, as and when needed, and I am pleased to say that her headaches went away and stayed away.

Let me share what Karen wrote at the time about her experience of working with me for help with her headaches:

"Five months ago a friend asked me to make an appointment with Emma to try and help with my daily headache problem, but I'd always had headaches and I was resigned to it being my lot in life. In fact, I'd been told many years before by my GP that I just had to learn to live with them. So in a very negative frame of mind, I booked my first session thinking... 'two hours, no way, it would all be over in twenty minutes and I'd be on my way home.'

Then, I met Emma...

Twenty minutes turned into the allotted two hours and things had been shared that I never thought I would be able to discuss with anyone, ever. I left that first meeting feeling lighter and just a tiny bit optimistic. Over the last five months, I've been on a journey with Emma guiding me along the way. When my headaches were down to two or three a week, I was very excited and happy but Emma wasn't—she was going for zero tolerance—and with trust, chat and lots and lots of laughter, we've finally got there!"

ANN

Ann came to see me after having been recommended by Arthur's mum, Laura. They'd sat at the swimming pool chatting and, as I imagine the scenario, Ann would have mentioned her migraines, Laura perhaps responded with how Arthur's had been helped with homeopathy, and one thing led to another.

Ann was sixty-three when we met and she told me that her only issue was migraines. They'd started around age sixteen—around the time of her first period—and had continued unabated since then. Other than the migraines, she stated that everything else was fine and she had a happy home and family life. The migraines, however, stopped her from doing what she wanted to do. She would usually have between two and four per month and they were severe enough that the pain could make her nauseous. She said she managed them to a degree, using a combined approach of Sumatriptan nasal spray and Amitriptyline daily, with painkillers on top, if needed.

She described the way she experienced her migraine headaches this way: 'It's a pulsating, throbbing pain. They can be anywhere in my head. They're worse for sunlight and noise. I'm not good with noise when I've got a headache, though generally I don't like quiet. Heat triggers them—I'm not good with hot, hot weather (around 19°C is enough). If I drink alcohol, that will also give me a migraine. For example, if I've been to a funfair on a warm day, I'll probably get one. They tend to last two days, but it can be three and I can be sick quite a few times with them.' In addition, she'd sometimes experience a burping sensation with the migraine, which is something we might call a Strange, Rare or Peculiar (SRP) symptom, meaning most people with headaches or migraines wouldn't experience this. Ann also had some digestive symptoms—eating could make the headaches worse—and sometimes constipation accompanied them. Finally, she commented that her sleep was not very good and she would periodically wake up at two a.m.

When asked to describe herself, Ann said, 'I'm a busy person, optimistic, just a granny and a mum. I like keeping home and cooking and caring for the farm animals.' I noted that she was always looking after other people—the grandchildren, her children, her husband. She liked things organised and enjoyed being busy.

After talking with Ann and working on her case, I felt Calcium carbonicum might work well for her as so many of her seemingly unconnected symptoms were included in this remedy's description: her tendency to want to be organised and busy; the frequent waking up at two a.m.; the burping while experiencing the headaches; and issues with heat, noise and light. The fact that details such as these are found in the *Materia Medica* books is quite incredible and still causes me to marvel at the genius of those who wrote these texts and discovered exactly what homeopathic medicines can assist with. I asked Ann to take the Calc carb as a split dose—one to be taken on the first evening and another on the second evening—with instructions to repeat in two weeks if she experienced no change.

We met six weeks later and Ann told me she was feeling so much better. She'd only had two headaches/migraines in that time. Not only had they reduced in frequency, but the intensity was also much diminished. On one occasion, she'd only had to use one spray of the Sumatriptan, which was unusual; she said normally she would need to use much more than this. The other occurrence she reported was more like a headache than a migraine and lasted only a day, where typically, it would have stayed for two to three.

At our second follow-up five weeks later, Ann told me:

"It's wonderful, absolutely wonderful. I took two tablets a month ago, only had one headache... not even a bad-bad one. I took two Paracetamols, where normally I'd have to take three lots of two, and the following day it had gone. Normally it would last two to three days and I would have had to take a nasal spray too. I've been with the children, had really busy days and it's also been really hot and I've been fine, which I wouldn't have expected. I'm also not feeling sick on a morning. I'm feeling so good. I don't think I realised how bad it was until I felt better. I really can't thank you enough. Such a worthwhile thing to have done. I've had the headaches for so long—basically all my life."

I've had other clients tell me the same thing—we often don't realise how bad things are until we no longer have to deal with them.

It was two years since we'd last met when I contacted Ann to seek permission to use her case in this book. She told me that the headaches had gradually returned over time and, though not as frequent or severe, they could still be intense. We spoke for a while, discussing her current symptoms and I sent more of the Calc carb to her with advice on when to take it. In a short time she improved. I encouraged her to remain on the remedy for two months (taken at monthly intervals) and Ann was happy with this. If they return in the future, we'll work to increase her health and reduce the headaches once again.

I asked her to put into words how working with homeopathy was for her and she said:

"A huge thank you for all your help sorting me out. Such a great result so far which has improved the quality of my life enormously. Thanks again."

Homeopathy isn't a miracle cure and it isn't always a quick fix. Ann had suffered with her migraine headaches for over forty years when we met. As I mentioned earlier in this text, one rule of thumb is that it may take a month for every year that it's been an issue for things to resolve. For Ann, this was smashed here. Though it may have been helpful for her to continue working with homeopathy for a little longer, I usually leave that decision to the client. We can schedule a follow-up in a few weeks, a few months or for longer down the line. Alternatively, people can get in touch as and when needed. That said, it's definitely worth having a follow-up consultation if you've had great results and then things slip back a bit. Chances are good that we can get back on the right track fairly quickly and easily once again.

2

Respiratory Issues

Using homeopathy for coughs, colds and 'flu-like symptoms is often one of the ways in which people start using it, and the first aid kits have several medicines that can help in these instances. As with anything, respiratory issues can be chronic or acute and I'll share a bit of both in this section. The first case is of an acute ailment (croup) that came on suddenly for my daughter. Here I focus more on the *symptoms* of the croup—how it started, what made it better or worse—than the bigger picture of who the person was that had the croup. In the two following cases—that of Claire and Kay—the key to finding a successful remedy was gaining an understanding of who they were as individuals, as well as understanding the symptoms they were experiencing.

Isla

My daughter Isla developed croup at the age of two. I'd never encountered croup before, so when her symptoms appeared late one evening I was concerned and considered calling for an ambulance or taking her to A&E. However, before I did either, I made one quick call to the Homeopathic Helpline.[1] Looking back, I should have figured out the homeopathic medicine myself, but I was in fearful mother mode and couldn't think straight at the time. It can be hard to prescribe for our families and even harder to self-prescribe. Our families can sometimes be too close to us for us to see a clear picture, and taking an objective look at ourselves isn't always easy either.

So I phoned for help and described my daughter's symptoms to Francis, the homeopath who answered the phone. After listening for a short time, he noted that Isla and I had been out during a crisp, blustery day in December and he recommended a medicine which mentioned a cold, dry wind as a common trigger factor. The timing of the symptoms, coming on specifically around midnight, was also highly relevant. Francis suggested a high potency of Aconite and fortunately I had that medicine in my home kit, so I gave a dose of it to Isla.

Aconite

Less than ten minutes later, Isla was sound asleep in my bed as if nothing had happened. She was breathing normally, her coughing was gone and her temperature had reduced. It felt like a miracle but of course it's not; it's just homeopathy at its best. The remedy needed repeating several times the next day, but in terms of speed of response, it was a beautiful illustration of how quickly homeopathy can act.

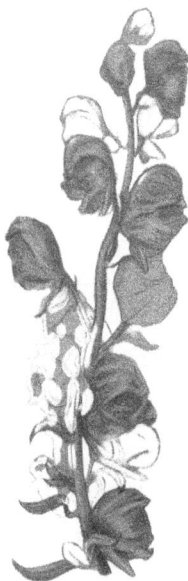

CLAIRE

Claire first sought help when she was going through a stressful period at work. She was thirty-nine at the time and had been dealing with asthma since the age of eight, when she was diagnosed by a physician.

Claire told me that her grandma, whom she had lived with for the first two years of her life, had died when Claire was eight. Ever since her death, if she was in a stressful situation, she would have an asthma flare-up, though at other times the breathing challenges might also appear out of nowhere. She'd been using an inhaler since her initial diagnosis and if she didn't use it, the symptoms would get worse. If she was cold, she might get really 'wheezy' and if she thought of work and allowed herself to get into a negative headspace about it, her breathing would get a lot worse too. Claire also described something else fairly new—different from the way she'd experienced stressful situations in the past—a fight or flight sensation which led to a feeling 'almost like I'm an animal being hunted, like I'm waiting for what's coming but I won't know what it is until it happens.' Following this, she would experience an itchy, irritating cough-like sensation all along her windpipe and slightly into her lungs, which at times felt 'like a constant, irritating tickle.'

In describing herself, Claire told me her peripheral vision is acute and she is highly in touch with her intuition and gut feelings, both of which are very strong. She relished being outdoors at competitive events, though she said she was probably one of the least competitive people there. She mainly entered into them because she enjoyed being out in nature and loved interacting with and encouraging others.

At the time we met, her lungs felt especially irritated at work; she would get that itching sensation in them and have to use her Ventolin inhaler a lot during the day just to feel comfortable. She added that she was awaiting a meeting regarding a grievance she had just brought to management against her boss, telling me, 'My office has a massive open-plan floor and my manager moved my desk so that I was in the open on a floor of two hundred and fifty people, with my boss positioned directly behind me in a clear line of sight. It's all very disjointed. I can't see or hear my team. I was the only manager not sat near their team but my boss insisted on having me at that desk. I felt monitored, constantly watched, feeling as if I was being hunted. It's like sticking a deer in an open field and giving someone a rifle. I hate the position of it, I don't feel connected to the team and it's very uncomfortable. I feel like my boss is waiting for an opportunity for me to screw up on something.' Claire said she knew that of the five other women on the fully-female senior leadership team, everyone had the same Myers Briggs personality profile except her, and that, 'I knew I was a non-fit and the whole experience felt crippling.'

Taking into account the picked-on, hunted feeling that Claire was experiencing, along with her breathing difficulties and love of movement, connection and being part of a group, after working on her case, I recommended a medicine made from the hair of the fallow deer, Dama dama, in a relatively high potency, to be taken in two doses. I'd like to stress that just because someone mentions a specific animal, it doesn't mean they're going to be given a homeopathic medicine from that animal. In fact, it's fairly uncommon to do that. But occasionally, there is a beautiful match and that was certainly the case here.

We met again after a month and Claire told me she'd had a difficult meeting regarding her grievance, but the stressful work environment she'd described in our last session was no longer relevant as she'd now left that role. She felt that this was a pivotal point in her life and mentioned that, while she had no idea where she was going, she was feeling excited about what was ahead. The physical sensations and stress were still a significant challenge for her, though her breathing was a lot better. She told me that the remedy had really helped and that she'd seen her breathing change quickly. On a mental and emotional front, she'd started seeing friends again and was happy to be back in touch with people.

Although weary from the experience she'd gone through at work, she was looking forward to a new role with a different organisation. There were also some self-confidence doubts (unsurprising with the stress of leaving her job) and we repeated the previous remedy.

Claire later wrote the following note to me:

"Hi Emma, I just wanted to say a huge thank you! I've never recovered quicker from stress-related asthma. I've gone from using my inhaler two to three times a day to twice in seven weeks! Additionally, I've found our conversations (usually me off-loading my thoughts) very helpful. Having the ability to talk through life's challenges and the circle of thoughts which can sometimes plague me daily, with your calming suggestions and amazing listening skills, I have moved forward successfully through a very difficult period. Amazingly, my lungs no longer have the constant itch, my breathing has calmed and overall I feel better! Genuine many thanks."

We met twice more in the years to come, both times when Claire was making potentially life-changing decisions. When thinking about the choices she had to make, she felt chest tightness once again—though not as badly as when we'd first talked—along with anxiety, which had also returned. She was experiencing the hunted feeling, too, like she knew something was going to happen, anticipating that whatever it was, it wasn't going to be great. It was all similar to the stress she had had with work and she simply didn't want to feel this way anymore. Claire was clear that she wanted to feel a sense of calm, a stillness within, as much as possible but was currently feeling drained, with the energy being taken out of her.

While the intensity was less than the time we first met, the symptoms she was experiencing were very similar to those discussed in our initial session. So, since she'd had such positive results the last time, I was encouraged that a repeat of the same remedy may well help her again. I suggested we repeat the Dama dama at a higher potency and if there was no change in two weeks, she should repeat the medicine with a single dose then. Once again this helped both her physical and emotional symptoms to improve.

When discussing sharing her story in this book, Claire wrote to me about our follow-up sessions to say:

"In relation to our meeting in 2021, I believe that once you have had the feeling of anxiety and how it displays itself within the body, when it happens again on a level that isn't fleeting, so more prolonged and intense, the need to act is there. There was no reservation in coming to see you, Em, and doing so before I got into a situation that felt unmanageable was important to me. This time the situation was beyond workplace bullying, it was the global impact of a 'pandemic' and the reactions of humanity, including my place of work.

During our conversation you said something which has stayed with me and will do for life. You said how I was feeling may have been justified. The impact of this one line and a remedy set me on a journey that changed my life for the better. It's so easy to think that how you feel is a problem that you've brought on, when in actual fact life circumstances can be so profound that your feeling of being 'hunted' and marginalised was in this case justified.

Sitting on a bench in the open air with birdsong all around grounded me and after our meeting my thoughts of what is truly important were compounded. Changing my life direction has been rewarding and you have been part of that journey. I'm living in an uneasy paradise, but the freedom is worth the material and financial sacrifice. Thank you for hearing me and prescribing accordingly."

KAY

Kay was fifty-eight when we met in late 2022. Her sinus issues—the reason she came to see me—had begun in January 2017, more than five years earlier. It had started when Kay had been ill with 'flu and then sinusitis and her sinuses had never been clear since. At this point, Kay said her Ear, Nose and Throat (ENT) Consultant was more concerned with her ears and had almost given up on the sinuses, saying nothing more could be done about them.

She described her symptoms as follows: 'Loss of smell and taste due to chronic sinusitis. A massive build-up of yellow mucus all day every day. Constantly clearing my nose and throat and sounding nasal when speaking.' In addition, her ears would 'get sticky'. As a child, she was always having problems with her hearing and recalled being asked to go for a hearing test by her school teacher. Now, she would still get a build-up of wax, which she'd often have to have flushed out. She'd actually been diagnosed with 'glue ear' a while ago. Her sinus symptoms were the worst at night and her sleep was disturbed as a result. She woke up a lot with dried mucus in her nose and often upon waking, she would find that she had dripped mucus on the pillow and the sheets. Close to midday things would get a little easier but by mid-afternoon, they'd get worse again.

Kay told me how she loved to travel, enjoyed teaching Pilates, did remedial massage therapy, used to teach in a specialist school and loved being creative. She was fun-loving, enjoyed having family around and wanted to be free. 'What does free mean?' I asked. I ask questions like this because I'm always conscious that it's easy to hear words and think I know what someone means but we are all so different—we can say the same words and mean very different things because of the unique ways each of us experiences the world around us.

For Kay, free meant 'free to move, to move around, to make my own choices, freedom of being me, not having to sort other people. Having my own space.' She liked to be in the sun, to swim in the sea and in cold water. She used to run marathons and loved distance runs but sadly had to give it all up—first due to the 'flu and then a hamstring injury. She didn't have many fears but wasn't a fan of small, crowded, noisy spaces, which made her feel like she needed to escape.

Given all she shared with me, I suggested Tuberculinum, a homeopathic medicine that has been used for many years, in a mid to high potency. I asked her to take two doses, one the first night and one the second, and then repeat if there'd been no change in two weeks.

We met four weeks later. Kay had noted some significant changes in terms of her symptoms. She was encouraged by the fact that, although nothing major had changed with her sense of smell, she'd actually been able to smell a toasty cooking recently. She was also sleeping better as she wasn't waking up so much in the night to unblock her nose. Since our first session, she'd had a nasal examination with a camera that confirmed damage in the olfactory nerve, but she still refused to believe that she'd never smell again. When we initially met, Kay joked that she had wondered about buying shares in Kleenex due to the number of tissues she was using—nearly thirty a day. At this first follow-up, she was now only using three tissues a day—a vast reduction in snot! Talking further about how things had changed, she said that before she started working with homeopathy there were times when she would have described her symptoms as ten out of ten in terms of severity; by our second session she rated them at a two.

We continued with the same remedy to take again and repeat in two weeks. At the next follow-up appointment, we increased the potency because, although she'd seen continued improvements with the lower potency, it seemed to 'run out' sooner than I would have liked. Also, she'd had an allergy test which had found that dust mites were an issue and this was a challenge at one of the places she worked. Interestingly, research suggests that the use of dust mite in homeopathic potency may help those who have a dust mite allergy (particularly of note is a published study by Dr Jonathan Hardy, done in his fourth year of medical school[2]). I'd also seen the remedy be very helpful myself each time I'd used it, so I gave it to Kay, and it was no different; it helped her too.

Meeting again in June 2023, she told me she felt an eighty-five percent improvement in her symptoms. Her ears were clear, her hearing test results were good, she no longer had scabs inside her nose, she was down to just one tissue during the night, she was sleeping well on the whole and she had been discharged from her consultant. There were still no changes in taste and smell, but she was really pleased with the improvements so far. I had to laugh at the end of the consultation as we were discussing the Greek Islands. I asked where her favourite one was and she responded, 'I don't know, I need to go to more of them to decide.' For me, it was further confirmation that Tuberculinum was a good match for her—people who match the Tuberculinum picture love to travel!

By now, Kay had an awareness of when she needed to repeat her remedy, so we no longer went with a two-week schedule. She simply repeated it when her symptoms seemed to slip back a little and there was more snot going on for her. I always like to get to this stage, when the client can repeat when needed instead of according to a set plan, because listening to our body and having the tools to respond feels to be so key in any healing process.

By July 2023, seven months into working with Kay, her ears were still clear and she no longer needed any tissues at night. There were still no significant changes in her smell and taste, though she had sensed that something was different when she was in the kitchen. Dust mite-wise, things were much better, although she could tell if she was somewhere particularly dusty. On waking, she would cough to clear her throat but wouldn't have to do anything else after that. In terms of her hearing, she couldn't believe it—she'd never known her hearing to be so good for so long. There was no stickiness, no popping or crackly sounds. Kay now rated her improvements in the ninety percent area and said, 'Even if it doesn't get better than this, this is amazing.' She still believed she would get her smell back.

Kay and I last met in September 2023, and she continued to be happy with her progress. She rated it as a ninety-nine percent improvement from when we started working together ten months previously. Excitingly, Kay also told me that her smell was finally coming back. In the last three days, she'd smelt onion, cauliflower, mint, washing powder and a man's fragrance. She said, 'I can't believe it—these last few days have been a real breakthrough. I can even feel the air as I breathe through my nose now.' She was back out running and felt like she was 'in control' of her breath. There was no cough and her hearing was absolutely fine. She'd recently returned from holiday and while normally a flight would set her ears off and she'd struggle for days after it, there was not a single issue this time. When I contacted Kay in December 2023 to ask for permission to use her story in this book, she told me she had last taken the remedy in the middle of October and remained well.

What a privilege it is to walk alongside people, to see the changes that happen for them—not to do it *for* them but to *support* them, bringing what I know to the table along with whatever they're doing as we work together. Seeing results like this always makes me so grateful that I'm doing what I do. One of my bugbears is that there are so many people needlessly suffering. Kay had spent nearly six years being ill and, despite two operations, was still 'almost drowning' in mucus daily, with an official message from conventional medical practitioners of, 'There's nothing more we can do.' It turned out that there *was* something she could do—and Kay did it.

3

Digestive Issues

Many of us experience challenges with digestion at different points in our lives, perhaps feeling temporarily sick or nauseous, as described in Ophelia's case below; or having a longer-lasting issue, as was the case with Erik; or we may experience more than one issue—of which digestion is only a part—which is what happened with Maayan. Maayan's story is featured in the Multiple Issues section—she initially came to see me for help with her anxiety and headaches along with her digestive health. It's worth noting that homeopathy kits have some wonderful medicines to support minor ailments in the area of digestion, however if symptoms are longer-lasting, a professional homeopath may be a good port of call.

Erik

Erik was seven when we first met. I've also worked with both of his brothers, Arthur and Ralf, as well as his mum Laura—their cases are also detailed in this book. Erik's reason for seeing me was his slow digestion—he'd frequently struggled with constipation and had done so since being very young. It got worse when he started school because he was too nervous to use the toilet there. His tummy would distend and he could get to the point where he would have an accident because he'd been holding it in for so long. He might empty his bowels every two days, though sometimes it would be every three to four. When he finally did have a bowel movement, his mum described it as 'an extraordinary poo, like the size of his arm.'

I asked Erik's mum about his personality, likes and dislikes, habits, etc. According to her, he had high energy and was always busy, occupied, on the go, doing things. She said he was a bit of a performer—he ran around shouting a lot and he liked to do dances and invent funny songs. When bored, he might go around annoying others—jumping on their back, then running off and laughing, for example. He loved pulling pranks (he had fake dog poo that ended up in someone's bed a lot!) and adored April Fool's Day. Erik also showed a lot of creativity and had recently written a comic book with his big brother. He was scared of dark places, especially at night. He wasn't keen on drinking and didn't eat a lot, mostly enjoying fruits. He felt better by the sea. As a baby, he was sensitive about his feet and didn't want to wear shoes, going barefoot whenever possible. When I asked what he wanted to be when he was older, he told me, 'If I was grown up tomorrow, for a job I'd do gardening or curate video games. I'd love to live in a log cabin in a "whole farm" next to a lake with loads of fish.'

Socially, he was outgoing and well-liked—his school report stated he had a lovely personality, got along with everyone and was a good friend. He liked to follow the rules, especially at school. His mum mentioned that when his teacher thought he had been naughty and told him so, he would never answer back. Although he didn't often stand up for himself, he would stand up for what's right—if something happened that he didn't feel was just, he could be very indignant. He was also very empathic. He tended to be protective of his older brother and was really good at anticipating situations that might cause him trouble. For example, if he saw a dog ahead, he'd run to be with his brother who doesn't like dogs. And if someone at school was hurt, or if his siblings were upset, he'd be the first to go and help them.

I initially gave Erik a medicine that didn't help and some of his mental/emotional symptoms intensified, so when we met for his follow-up consultation, I went back to the drawing board. When I reviewed the details of his case, I again noted his mischievous side, constant desire to be busy and on the go, as well as the symptom of constipation. This time, I decided to give Lycopodium in a moderately high potency, which seemed to fit his physical symptoms particularly well. His mum was astounded by the result. Here's what she wrote to me:

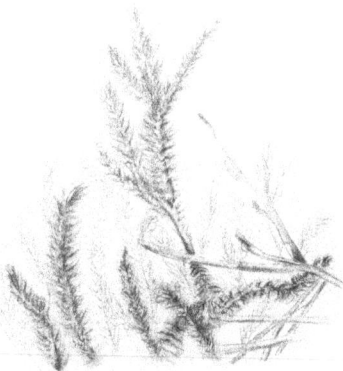

Lycopodium

> *"Erik is like a different child!! He hasn't withheld a poo since we saw you. He's very regular and has an appetite for the first time in his life. He has a real enthusiasm for eating now and he's always saying that he's hungry, which is something he never did before. He looks much healthier—a bit more flesh in his face and less pale. I can't believe it. Homeopathy wins again!! Thanks so much!"*

I love a happy result in clinic—it makes all the work so worthwhile.

OPHELIA

When I travel I tend to take a homeopathy kit with me, and while my daughter and I were in Greece in summer 2023, it was no different. We dipped into our Helios Homeopathy 36 medicine kit frequently for too much sun, insect bites, headaches and more.

On the penultimate day of our trip, we were chatting to a waitress in our hotel and, after asking out of politeness how she was, she mentioned her head and stomach didn't feel good. I replied that I hoped she felt better soon. 'Mum,' urged my daughter, 'go and ask if you can help her. She's so lovely and you could give her something from the kit.'

Back when I graduated, I'd have been running after her, asking if I could help. I wanted to shout to the whole world about homeopathy back then. Now I'm far quieter about what I do, but my daughter was right—the waitress *had* been really lovely with us during our stay and if I could help, it would be a nice way to thank her for all her care. With the help of another waitress to translate, I asked Ophelia to describe her symptoms. She told me she was feeling dizzy and nauseous and after a little more information, I left her with a few Nux vomica tablets in an envelope as this really felt to match what she was describing. She was so grateful that we'd tried to help her and insisted on giving us each a drink from the bar as a thank you.

The first remedy given may not be the perfect match, in which case you may need to change the medicine, repeat it or change the potency. With that in mind, I said I'd pop back in about forty-five minutes, before we got the bus into town for our final night out. When we called in, Ophelia told us she felt great—her symptoms had cleared after taking the remedy once. I suggested that she repeat it if she felt that her symptoms were returning but, unless that happened, there was no need to take it again. She was so happy to be feeling better and it was lovely to be able to show our gratitude for this lovely lady who had taken such good care of us.

4

SKIN COMPLAINTS

Skin complaints can sound like such a simple thing to 'fix'—apply a cream and the symptom 'goes'—but with conditions like eczema, that fix isn't always so easy. Sure, more cream or a medication taken indefinitely is one potential solution, but you can often find yourself over time having to use a stronger and stronger cream (for example, a steroid cream) to keep the issue 'under control.' This section includes four cases that demonstrate longer-term skin challenges—for some of these clients, their symptoms had been around for a few months but with others, a few decades.

When I teach on my *Introduction to Homeopathy* courses, I like to share an analogy—that of a warning light on a car. When the warning light comes on, we can either remove the light and pretend there isn't a problem or we can investigate further. When we apply a cream or suppress a symptom, it's almost like removing our own warning light because our symptoms are an external expression of an underlying problem—an imbalance that needs our attention. This is why, in the homeopathic world, we're as likely to be curious about the 'you' that is experiencing the symptoms as we are about the symptoms themselves. Ideally, knowing both of these things will lead us to give a homeopathic medicine that not only sees your symptoms improve but helps you better navigate life too.

While homeopathy kits contain medicines that are brilliant at helping common skin issues like insect bites, stings, cuts, grazes and bruising resolve more quickly, longer-lasting symptoms often require the skill of matching a remedy to the person, as we'll see in the cases in this section.

Juliet

I first met Juliet at the end of January 2023. She described to me how she'd had eczema for quite some time on her fingers but never on her face or hands, which is where it was now.

Juliet described her new symptoms as red, inflamed, itchy and dry skin which would then flake off, especially on her eyelids. It had also appeared on the back of her hands and would weep clear fluid. Occasionally, the skin would become infected and then the weepy discharge would be a yellowish colour. When her itching was bad, she would rub her hands on anything—her trousers, bathroom towels or bed sheets—to get relief. She mentioned that she'd had a similar bout when her daughter was born sixteen years earlier, which lasted for about six months, though it went away when she cut out gluten. This time, she'd also cut out gluten for the last six months but it hadn't made a difference. Nothing made her symptoms better apart from antihistamines.

When I asked her to tell me about herself, she described to me how she had always liked her work as a pharmacy dispenser since she fell into it about twenty years ago. As a child she was quiet and socially awkward at times.

I also asked her if there was anything particular happening in her life when this new bout started. Juliet told me that just over two years ago, her aunt and uncle had died within weeks of each other from Covid and then her cousin's partner passed away. There were also additional stresses within the family—more health challenges that were going on around her.

This led me to ask her how she coped with stress. This is an aspect of life that affects us all so differently, so knowing how someone responds to life's pressures may help me in the quest to find a matching homeopathic medicine. As to how Juliet handled stress, she said, 'I can get short-tempered. I can get overwhelmed.' She added, 'My mum would probably say I get too stressed about things I don't need to. My partner says I worry too much—I worry about things that I don't know will happen.'

She also shared that she had recently experienced some mild depression, as well as pre-menstrual syndrome (PMS). The depression wasn't to the point that it was hard to function—she was still walking the dog and taking her daughter to school—but she did feel listless and couldn't be bothered to do normal things like cook or do household chores. She loved to read, consuming two to three books a week but when depressed, she didn't read for weeks at a time. About six weeks prior, she had gone to the doctor, who gave her ten milligrams of Citalopram to take daily and she was feeling okay now.

Juliet had also seen her GP for her skin issues. Dermatitis was the physician's diagnosis and she'd been given steroid creams for it. She was also prescribed a steroid nasal spray, to be used for six weeks, because in addition to her skin flare-up, her nose had been blocked too. Regarding her nose, Juliet said it was worse when the heating was on and when she was lying down. She definitely felt better when she was outdoors.

Bearing in mind Juliet's family losses, her reserved nature, her desire to stay occupied—whether that be with the work she enjoyed, walking or reading—and her skin symptoms, I gave a high potency of Natrum muriaticum, which is a polychrest (or often-used homeopathic medicine) to take twice and then if there was no change, to repeat in two weeks' time.

We met for a follow-up two months later and she said her skin had improved a lot just two weeks after our first meeting. It had already started clearing before she took the second round of tablets, first on her hands (which were almost back to normal now) and then on her face. Her itching had gone from a ten out of ten down to a four. She went on to say that if she was grooming or feeding their family horse, it would itch a bit but after she washed her hands, it would stop. Her 'blocked-up nose' had disappeared, she said: 'After about two weeks, I got up one day and realised it wasn't blocked anymore.' Juliet also told me that she wasn't constantly needing to rub her hands on anything for relief from the itching.

She added that, as her skin cleared, she'd had a few cold sores pop up. This wasn't anything new—she'd had them for ages—however, they were smaller than usual and not even very noticeable, just sore. This is termed a 'return of old symptoms'[1] in homeopathy and is actually a good sign. A return of old symptoms, typically in reverse order of their occurrence in our lives, is one of Hering's Laws of Cure in homeopathy and a sign of a well-matched medicine. An old symptom (for example, Juliet's cold sores) can reappear for a short time if it has been suppressed in some way, often by taking conventional medicine. It typically goes away after a repeat of the homeopathic remedy, as it did in this case.

Juliet's mood was so much better that she told me she kept forgetting to take her Citalopram. She had even had her period the week prior to when we met but unlike before, when she used to experience PMS, she didn't even notice her period was coming until it arrived. Because Juliet's improvements had been so significant, I decided the best response for now was to wait, rather than repeat the Nat mur, and check in on her progress at our next meeting.

We met again a month later and Juliet told me that, although she'd just attended her third funeral in three weeks, she was coping well. Aside from a small patch of eczema under her eye, her skin was doing fine. Though there was obviously a lot of sadness with the new family losses she had experienced, her mood was otherwise stable. Her blocked nose was also clear, sometimes feeling a little stuffy if the heating was on but aside from that, all was good. She couldn't remember the last time she felt the need to rub her hands on anything and wasn't scratching at night, which had been the case earlier. She now rated her overall skin symptoms at a one or two out of ten, instead of the ten out of ten itching and discomfort she'd had before. I advised her to repeat the remedy if her symptoms got worse and to get in touch if that didn't help.

When I messaged Juliet in October 2023 to ask about using her case in the book, she said, 'It's fine to include my story in the book. I'm still pretty much eczema-free!'

Steve

Steve, my partner, had a cyst on his head when we met. Never having encountered homeopathy before, he happily followed the conventional medical route to explore the options and I wasn't rushing forward to volunteer alternative solutions.

When I first graduated, I was so eager and wanted to help everyone. Looking back, I am reminded of the 'Jesus man' who stands on a street in our town on busy days, handing out cards and telling people that Jesus loves them. Like the 'Jesus man', I was passionate and on a mission. I wasn't exactly running up to people and telling them I could save them, but honestly, I wasn't far off. Now, older and a bit wiser, I no longer rush forward volunteering my services, so with Steve I sat back as he took his course of antibiotics. And another. And no change.

By this point, he'd had another consultation with a GP. Her recommendation was another course of antibiotics and, if there was still no change, she'd slice the cyst open, gouge around in it and clear it out. He might be left with a bald patch where the cyst was but otherwise, it would all be sorted. Thinking back, this was not unlike my horse's eye disease experience—remove the diseased bit and away we go. Steve was less than keen. I'm not sure if it was the word 'gouge' in connection with his scalp or the threat of potential baldness that really bothered him, but seeing his reticence around the process, I quietly mentioned that if he wanted to tell me a bit more about the symptoms, I could see if there was a homeopathic medicine that might help. By that stage, he was eager to see if homeopathy could make a difference.

The cyst was red, very hot, throbbing and painful to touch, which fit the picture of Belladonna, a medicine made from the deadly nightshade plant of the same name. I went with a medium to high potency to fit the intensity of the cyst's symptoms.

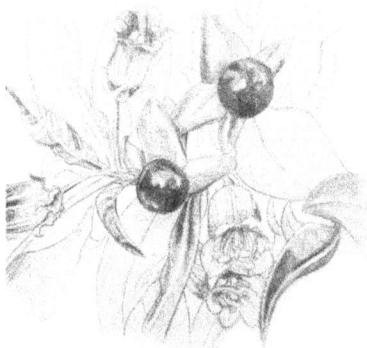

Belladonna is particularly interesting in many ways and a great example of how Hahnemann harnessed the healing

Belladonna

power of poisonous plants and other toxic substances. Homeopathic medicines are extremely safe and are highly diluted, energetic substances. Once they have gone through this process of dilution and succussion (shaking), there is nothing of the original source material left in most of the potencies that we use within our work. This is baffling to some. The 'logical' argument goes that if there is nothing left of the original material, then how can it possibly do anything to help a person get well? I can't tell you exactly how it works—many fabulous researchers are working on that question and getting closer to a definitive answer—though what I *can* tell you is that the homeopathic dilution and succussion process makes a potent healing remedy when matched to the symptoms correctly.

After Steve had taken the Belladonna several times, the pain, redness and heat were significantly reduced but the cyst itself was still very much there. At this stage, we started to alternate Hepar sulph with Silica. Hepar sulph has earned a reputation in some homeopathic circles as 'the homeopathic antibiotic', and while I want to steer you away from a 'this for that' concept of homeopathy, it's a good one to check out when there is some kind of infection. If it fits with what's going on, it can be a wonderful medicine to use but it's important to note that choosing a well-matched homeopathic remedy is far more than 'if I have an infection, I'll take Hepar sulph.' I have at least twenty-five medicines mentioned in my repertory under 'Head, cysts' and one hundred and fifty-four under 'Skin, cysts' so, as ever, we need to make sure the symptoms fit.

Silica is a useful medicine for expelling foreign bodies, such as splinters. I've heard one tale of a jeweller taking Silica for another complaint and finding a tiny fragment of silver, which had been lodged in his nose for years, finally emerge. On this note, if you have a pacemaker, surgical pins or other foreign bodies internally that have been placed there for therapeutic use, don't take lots of Silica! Many homeopaths suggest avoiding the medicine entirely if their client has any of the above.

By repeating Hepar sulph and Silica for several days, Steve's cyst grew smaller each day. After a week or two, aside from the smallest lump, which could be mistaken for a teeny tiny spot, the cyst was pretty much unnoticeable unless you knew it was there. It has remained that way ever since.

It's been six years now and the cyst has never needed surgical intervention, nor required further antibiotics or other conventional medication—just three commonly used, readily available homeopathic medicines. It was a real privilege to be on hand to witness the changes as they happened.

JOHN

John was seventeen years old at the time of our first consultation. He had been given steroids for eczema in the past and was now experiencing topical steroid withdrawal (TSW).

His story is fairly typical for many with this skin ailment. He had allergies and eczema at age two, which improved massively with conventional treatment at the time, though it 'came back with a vengeance' when he was fifteen. The steroid cream initially worked brilliantly, but the eczema continued to return with less time in between flare-ups. At this point, it can be tempting to use stronger and stronger steroid creams, however, John and his mum realised that the steroids weren't really working all that well, given his eczema never resolved and was requiring higher and higher doses of medication. Longer term, it just didn't make sense to them to continue in this way, so John stopped the creams—and then went into full blown topical steroid withdrawal.

Now quite a few months into his TSW, John's skin where visible was mostly red, dry and flaky, with patches that were bleeding and oozing. At any one time, he could have these patches anywhere on his body. His palms were always clear but the backs of his hands and the ends of his fingers were red, inflamed and raw and his fingers were seeping. He said if he tapped a fingertip by mistake with his nail it was really sore. He also couldn't sleep for very long due to his discomfort. He had to change the sheets on his bed daily, as otherwise, 'I'd be lying in a pile of my own skin.' Bathing made the symptoms worse. Though the bath could feel relaxing while he was in it, afterwards his skin would dry out fast and he'd have to apply cream all over.

John itched intensely. He'd actually stopped going to school as he struggled with anxiety caused by the intense urge to scratch, which could spiral out of control into panic. He also found it so difficult to concentrate that it made things like taking exams impossible. Until the last few years, he'd described himself as very easy-going and sociable. Now, however, it took a lot of effort to make himself presentable to meet friends, and things he used to enjoy, such as playing rugby, made him so nervous they were no longer possible. He said it felt like torture to go through every day and that he 'wouldn't wish this condition on his worst enemy.' At this stage, he could no longer remember what it was like to be 'normal'. When I asked, 'What's the worst thing about it all?' he answered, 'Not feeling comfortable in my own skin.'

Given John's anxiety (which he experienced around both stressful events like exams and pleasurable events like playing rugby), lack of confidence and distinctive skin symptoms, along with his feeling better in the open air and other aspects he described, I gave a low potency of Graphites to be taken daily in water. Graphites can be a wonderful skin remedy when it fits the person and it seemed to fit both John and his symptoms well, so I was intrigued to see how he would get on with it.

We met again six weeks later and he told me he was definitely a lot better. Two weeks after he'd started taking the remedy, he was getting more sleep and was back at school part-time. The oozing on his skin had nearly stopped and he was changing his sheets every three days or so instead of daily. When we met the first time, he rated the itchiness at one hundred percent but was now rating it at fifty-five percent. Previously, it had been a lot worse in the early evening; now that no longer happened. Also, when he did feel the need to scratch, he didn't spiral out of control towards a panic attack. The reduction in the constant itching meant that he could live more normally, and subsequently his mental state was much more stable. He was seeing friends more often and he could be 'more bubbly' now. John's mum saw the change, too, mentioning that he was more like himself.

We next met eleven weeks after our initial session and John now reported that the itching was down to forty percent of what it was at the beginning. While he was still changing his bedsheets every three or four days, he told me this was because his standards had gone up, not because there hadn't been progress in this area. John was able to shower (which he hadn't been able to do before), his wrists were starting to look a lot less red and sore, the skin on his back had returned to normal and he wasn't waking up to scratch in the night. He was also now back at school full-time. As his skin continued to improve, he shared that he was feeling less self-conscious: 'My confidence has skyrocketed in the last month or so.' Finally, he was actually able to relax, something he realised he hadn't been able to do for so long due to the constant itching.

John still had some oozing on his fingers, which isn't uncommon. I sometimes see eczema reduce to a patch on someone's fingers or toes right before it 'leaves the body' altogether. Perhaps this is a strange concept if you're not used to homeopathic philosophy but it follows Hering's Law of Cure.[2] If you remember, the Law of Cure states that healing happens from above downwards, from inside to outwards, from the more central to more peripheral, from more important organs to less important ones and in the reverse order of disease appearance. While not every single case fits all of these aspects, the guidelines are useful in understanding our progress as we move towards a place of better health. When there is eczema everywhere, it is frequently seen to disappear from the more central areas of the body first and lastly from the more external areas of the body—exactly what was happening for John.

Six weeks later, John reported that things were steadily improving in most areas and we continued to increase the potency of the remedy.

Meeting after a further six weeks, John told me he'd experienced some setbacks but had bounced back nicely from them. He was now sleeping at least six hours a night and no longer needed a nap after school. His fingers were much better; there was no soreness and the skin wasn't raw. The skin on his legs was also much improved from last time. He recalled that in the past, he felt that in the areas that itched, his skin was somehow 'weaker', like he could easily damage it as he scratched; now he felt as if the skin was 'stronger' again. He was able to take both showers and baths and afterwards not have to put on as much cream; while before he was going through a tub of Epiderm a week, now it would last for three weeks. He was back playing rugby and enjoying it. In addition, John had had some alcohol—which used to cause an aggravation of his skin symptoms—and had no reaction from it. Finally, he noticed that his periods of feeling 'up' lasted much longer.

John's condition was so intense when he first came to me—he was in such a bad way both mentally and physically—so I was delighted with the progress he'd made. John's story continues and I'm very hopeful for his future.

LAURA

Laura was someone I worked with in a typical way that happens as a homeopath—first you see the children in clinic, then one or both of the parents at some point too. I see this happen a lot in my practice.

Laura was in her thirties when we first met, and consulted me for a skin problem that she'd had since her late teens. She described it as 'dry skin, little bubbles under the skin that would burst and sting, almost like eczema or psoriasis' that would flare up and down over time. When she was younger, the skin on her feet would ooze so badly that her socks would stick to her foot and she'd have to peel off the sock. It tended to be worse in winter, when constantly wearing socks, boots, etc. and better for being in open air in the warmer months, especially when she was on the beach. Now, in particular, it tended to flare up if she swam in a pool with her children, and if she swam consecutive weeks it could become stinging, throbbing and really sore, weeping with a clear, sticky excretion. At the time we met, it was only on her left foot, but she'd also had it on her hand at one time and was then diagnosed with contact dermatitis by a physician. At this point, she felt she'd 'tried nearly everything' to clear it and nothing so far had worked.

As happens with many complaints, it would be worse in times of stress. Laura's condition first started when she went through a time of worry and was having anxiety attacks about random things. She described herself as 'a bit nervous' and said she was quite shy and introverted, even grumpy and antisocial as a child, being so quiet that sometimes she didn't speak at all. She had a small circle of friends, didn't like group activities and was very much a homebody. She'd always felt fearful and vulnerable at school and was happiest with her family in her home environment.

Laura had always been claustrophobic—she didn't like busy or noisy spaces—to the point that she would choose the end seat of a row at the theatre so she could leave quickly if she needed to. She told me she liked to be cosy; she loved getting wrapped up in blankets and making dens as a kid. Interestingly, even though she was claustrophobic, she'd always loved cupboards under the stairs, seeking them out to have a look inside. She also loved the outdoors and would spend as much time in nature as possible. She remained anxious into her teen years and early twenties, however since her children were born, she no longer experienced anxiety saying, 'Whatever situation is thrown at me, I just deal with it. If they're happy and safe, I'm happy and safe.'

There were also other aspects of her personality that had shifted a bit from when she was a child. For example, she never used to fight back but would currently stand up for what she believed in. She said, 'I'm more aggressive. No, not the right word—I'm not as gentle as I was when I was younger. You've got to fight for your right in this world. I'm more forceful now.' In addition, Laura had always felt like an outsider but, as an adult, while she didn't want to follow the crowd, community was important to her.

Dolphins were her favourite animal but she preferred looking at them rather than being in the water. Interestingly, two years after she told me this, she had embraced wild swimming as enthusiastically as anyone I've ever met!

With Laura, the themes that came up in our discussion—a love of being cosy (but needing for it to be on her terms), the value she placed on caring for others and the way she talked about groups in regard to being in them or not—all had me thinking of a mammal remedy. I particularly took note of her love of cupboards, even more with the children around now, which intrigued me because of the claustrophobia. This was something of a polarity, two elements that were opposing, and I thought it might be fundamental to her case. Another polarity that I noticed was her shyness and caring nature combined with her ability to fight back when she really needed to. These were all clues to her possible remedy and

I selected Lac felinum, a homeopathic medicine made from cat's milk, in a medium potency.

We met five weeks later and Laura told me she was 'completely mind-blown' and that she'd never seen her skin that normal in twenty years. She said that within twenty-four hours, 'the thing on my foot had gone. It disappeared completely.' She told me her toe used to look as if it had been burnt but after the remedy, it was completely normal. It was all clear for a good few days then came back fairly suddenly across three toes. She waited two weeks, repeated the remedy and it disappeared completely again. It did return once more after being clear for a week, though not as angry or raw—just a bit dry and flaky. She mentioned she hadn't changed anything else, so the remedy was the only variable factor involved. She was amazed.

We repeated the medicine and spoke again a month later. The dermatitis had still not cleared fully, so I advised taking the remedy in a higher potency. Later, the problem had gone from her toes, but was back just a little under her foot, so I gave Lac felinum again in a slightly different potency, as well as in liquid form, to repeat as needed.

On contacting Laura about using her story in this book she said:

"The change was unbelievable. Up until taking the remedy, I'd been very wary about what I wore on my feet. And especially when going to the swimming pool, I'd wear swim socks to protect my skin. My dermatitis would flare up at times and was never completely clear. After taking the remedy it disappeared completely but then returned a few days later, although nowhere near as bad as before. After repeating the remedy, it cleared up completely once again, only to return once more, though even less so than before. And after using the recent drops once a day for a couple of weeks, it completely disappeared, no [more] flare ups and no irritation after pool swimming. I'd had this skin condition for the whole of my adult life—over twenty years! Thanks to Em and homeopathy, three years later, my skin is still completely clear. Magic!"

5

WOMEN'S HEALTH

(MENOPAUSE, PREGNANCY AND CONCEPTION)

I find that people often want to see a homeopath when they're going through times of change, whether that be emotional, mental or physical. For women, the desire to work through challenges with menstruation, menopause or pregnancy without conventional medications is a common reason for them to seek out complementary and alternative options. In this section, I'd like to share the stories of Caz, who worked with homeopathy during menopause, and Hara, who used homeopathy when she had fertility challenges.

CAZ

Caz had used homeopathy for many years. Initially she'd seen a homeopath, then gone on to use first aid/minor ailment homeopathic medicines on her own. She consulted me in January 2022, age fifty-four, for help with insomnia, hot flushes and night sweats that she'd had since the onset of menopause at age fifty-one.

Caz told me she was struggling but wasn't sure why—she had a healthy diet, exercised and had a positive outlook on life but even so, menopause 'hit me like a sledgehammer'. She reported a lack of energy, trouble sleeping, 'picking holes in myself' (being very self-critical) and a feeling of being overwhelmed. She also felt 'a bit weird at times—phased out' but finding it difficult to describe. She mentioned that when she was fifty-one, she was crying a lot and was emotionally more 'seesaw-y'. Now she was more level—'not on a good level but on a level somewhere.'

She'd always had a very regular, problem-free menstrual cycle and then two to three years before her periods stopped, she developed the worst pre-menstrual tension (PMT) that she'd had in years. Instead of 'feeling rubbish for two to three days' before her period, she would have 'ten days of feeling rubbish' before them.

When her periods stopped, she developed vasomotor symptoms and would wake with 'horrible palpitations in the middle of the night.' She told me she'd called the GP thinking there was something wrong with her heart but had felt he was very condescending towards her. He told her if she came in to the practice, he'd leave a prescription of Hormone Replacement Therapy (HRT) for her to collect, but didn't feel the need to see her in person. Not keen to take the medication, Caz decided to take some adaptogenic herbs to support her health. They'd worked a treat for a while for her sleep, though her PMT and energy levels were still a challenge.

When we met, Caz was having three or so hot flushes during the day, which she felt were manageable, but the night sweats were really hard. She'd wake boiling hot but then a few hours later feel shivery and dreadful. She also began experiencing 'fight or flight' symptoms and her sleep got even worse. Sometimes she would only sleep for one and a half hours a night, wake up warm and restless and then would be utterly sleepless until finally falling back to sleep around six or seven a.m. Caz said, 'If I could just get a good night's sleep, I could conquer the world.' She told me how 'everything felt crap'. She described the last three years as 'struggle after struggle' and was completely worn out.

Caz described herself as having a lot of tenacity and, while compassionate, she said it was with a bit more tough love than she used to have. She adored nature, was a constant seeker and was compelled to explore things in more depth. She didn't like the thought of rigidity, saying, 'I can't stagnate. I like to be flowing.' She was freedom-loving and desperate for change in the world. She was also creative in her work and felt like she was just getting going in terms of her career. Even though she felt so worn out, she was still enthusiastic and wanted the energy to be able to do the things she wanted to do. Things were admittedly difficult at the moment but in general, she said, 'I like being me.'

In Caz's case, there was a lot to take into account—hormonal changes, a desire to explore and travel, her creativity and sensitivity, her waking times, food desires, love of nature and dislike of summer and intense humid heat. Putting this all together, I selected the homeopathic medicine Sepia in a high potency, one a night for three nights, to be repeated in two weeks if there had been no change.

We met after six weeks and Caz told me she had improved a lot, even though she had experienced a lot of stress since she last saw me. While the symptoms had intensified a little on the second night of taking the remedy—'I felt as if all the crap was coming out of me'—on the third day, she felt a lot better. After two weeks, she'd repeated the medicine and said she felt the flushes had lessened, her nausea was much better and she was aware that her low mood was happening less. Spring was approaching and Caz noted, 'The light is returning,' which helped with her overall sense of well-being. Sleep was still an issue but now every second night she was sleeping quite well.

The seeker in Caz meant she also kept exploring ways to support her health on her own. She noticed that eating grains or high starchy vegetables for her evening meal would worsen her thermal activity. Sugar and beetroots during the day would increase the night sweats too. She would later suggest the book *The Glucose Goddess*[1] to me, having found the approach within it useful. I found it to be a helpful read as well and have gone on to recommend it to others since.

At this stage, we switched the remedy to a different potency of Sepia to be taken daily. After another month, Caz said that overall, she was quite a bit better. The thermal activity at night had absolutely gone and her sleep, while not perfect, was much improved. She was still being careful about what she ate in the evenings, which she felt had also helped. She told me she was no longer so self-critical, was doing yoga in the mornings and was overall achieving more in work and life.

At one point during our work together, Caz shared that her dad was dying. Since it was such a difficult time for her emotionally, I decided to change the medicine based on this new information, combined with the details given in her original consultation. We switched to Ignatia, to be taken daily, along with a low potency of cortisol to be taken occasionally. She then got back in touch with me before our next scheduled session because she had some acute symptoms of a badly blocked sinus with a headache, for which I suggested she take a few tablets of Natrum muriaticum as an acute remedy for those symptoms.

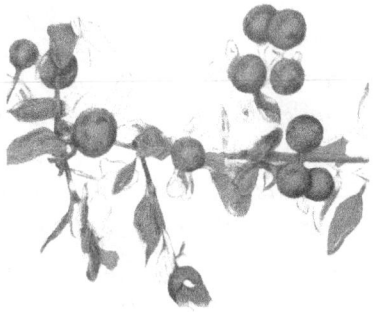

Ignatia

When we next met, Caz told me the Nat mur had worked a treat for the sinus and headache symptoms. She also described how, even though she felt emotionally drained in regard to her father's illness, she was feeling different. Within days of taking the Ignatia, she'd felt that it 'steadied me' stating, 'I think Ignatia is helping me be a bit more resolute. I have my moments but other people have also noticed how much better I am. I'm not so needy, not so out of control and I'm more resourceful. I have a lot of plans of what I want to do. I felt like I had no plans before and every day I was struggling. I don't feel like that now.'

Caz has continued to see me for various things, as well as generally supporting her overall health. One of the newest challenges she'd faced was a change in her eye health—not uncommon during menopause—for which she was taking some conventional medications in the form of eye drops from her optician, in addition to her homeopathic remedies. In a consultation in November 2023, Caz shared:

> "Thank you for that eye remedy—I had an eye examination recently and the health of my eyes is great. The vitreous fluid has pulled away from the back of the eye a little, which they said is normal with ageing, and I paid for a scan to find out how things are going. They said everything was really great. Seems like the remedy was fantastic. Previously I'd been described as having 'a cascade of floaters' and they would obscure my vision. I'd been told they're not going to go away but now I'm not aware of any of them. I took about half the bottle [it was a remedy to take daily] and something happened with it. I knew when it was time to stop and I stopped it, then the eye test confirmed things were going well. I feel like it really did give my eyes such a boost. I'm not noticing floaters—it's like they're just not there anymore."

In addition to using homeopathic medicines, Caz has a regimen that includes yoga, acupuncture, eating well, walking and getting outside. There is a saying that the best doctors are sunshine, air, exercise, water, diet, rest and laughter. I agree that those are great ways to support our health, and in my opinion, Caz partakes in all of these things well. I'm so grateful for Caz's innate curiosity, her readiness to explore additional ways to boost her own health and her willingness to have me on her team!

Hara

Hara is a homeopath herself and when she discovered I was writing this book, she offered to tell her own story of how homeopathy helped her conceive, carry and birth her children. I'm sure you'll agree, it's a pretty inspiring read and I'm grateful to her for allowing me to share it with you.

As a side note, I've personally seen homeopathy help several people conceive who've been trying for some time without success, though I would also say that I have colleagues who work much more with fertility challenges than I do. While I've pondered choosing a niche over the years, each time I realise how much I enjoy working with the variety of health challenges that I get to see in clinic and the different people I am privileged to walk alongside.

But enough chatting—let's dive in to Hara's wonderful story:

"The story of how my three children came into this world is a testament to the incredible power of homeopathy. After five long years of trying to conceive and a formal diagnosis of infertility, it was homeopathy that made the impossible possible, not just once but three times. Each of our babies was a deeply cherished dream, and homeopathy was the 'magic' that brought them into our lives.

Before turning to homeopathy, I explored various holistic treatment modalities like acupuncture, massage and herbal remedies, hoping to find a solution to our fertility struggles. However, it was only homeopathy that could address the delicate imbalances within my body and pave the way for healthy and viable pregnancies. With homeopathy, we were able to create the family we had always envisioned.

I happily travelled across North America to consult with a highly successful homeopath who was also a trained medical doctor. He prescribed Lachesis muta in low potency for my fertility chal-

lenges. In just four short months, I was pregnant and able to avoid harsh medical interventions.

The power of homeopathy didn't stop at conception. Throughout each pregnancy, I relied on homeopathy to manage various symptoms, ensuring that our children were nurtured and protected from the very beginning. Homeopathy even played a vital role in the birthing process, contributing to a successful and empowering experience each time. Recovery after delivery was also easier with the use of homeopathic medicines!

Our children have grown up in a world where homeopathy is the cornerstone of their healthcare (our pets too). They know no other form of medicine, and our family has wholeheartedly embraced this very easy holistic lifestyle by choice. Homeopathy is a brilliant system of medicine that empowers us to take control of our health challenges. It is safe, affordable, accessible, and remarkably effective, offering us a path to well-being that we embody fully.

In the world of homeopathy, we embrace the Latin motto 'Aude Sapere!'—dare to be wise. Our journey to parenthood has shown us that wisdom and healing can be found in the most unexpected places and, for us, that place is homeopathy. My story is one of hope, resilience and the boundless potential of natural medicine to shape our lives in extraordinary ways. Homeopathy has been our trusted companion on this remarkable journey of life, and we are forever grateful for its role in our world. Our family remains in touch with the homeopath who helped us with our fertility issues, and the relationship we have built over 15 years is special.

The story of my children's conception is just one powerful example of homeopathy's brilliance. I have been a homeopath for fifteen years and routinely witness life-changing results in my patients, from acute to chronic conditions, making it a beacon of hope in a world where many are in need, where our 'healthcare systems' often fall short. Every homeopath I know can convey the same sentiment. This natural system of medicine is becoming more popular around the world for a reason—because it works! I feel blessed to have found homeopathy and to be able to help others on their journey to good health, including those struggling with infertility!

One last thought: homeopathy has changed my family's life. As a parent, I feel I have given my children the greatest gift possible: empowerment over their healthcare choices. My children turn to homeopathy when needed, and having this system of medicine in their back pockets means they will prioritise it when raising their own families. We have given them the legacy of homeopathy, a gift that will continue to nourish and safeguard future generations."

6

ARTHRITIS AND JOINT COMPLAINTS

As with many of the conditions discussed in this book, homeopathy can be used both on an acute level for minor ailments and for longer term, more complex challenges too. Arnica montana, probably the best known homeopathic medicine, can be amazing for bruising, injuries and even exhaustion. If I was running a long distance race, I'd definitely have a small vial of Arnica in my pocket! Sometimes I jokingly refer to Arnica as 'our gateway drug' because it's one that people often get started with and it can end up hooking them on homeopathy for life. Other homeopathic medicines, such as Ruta graveolens and Rhus toxicodendron, which can work wonders on sprains and strains, fit this bill too.

In this section, you'll meet Liz, who has worked with homeopathy for years, and Diane, who was initially sceptical towards homeopathy before working with a homeopath, after which she started using it herself for minor ailments, and—as explained in her story here—then using homeopathy to assist in her recovery from surgery. I really like the way both stories weave their way between homeopathic and conventional interventions. Hopefully, you're getting a sense by now that it certainly doesn't have to be an 'either/or approach'!

Liz

Liz initially began working with homeopathy after being diagnosed in 2000 with rheumatoid arthritis (RA), an autoimmune disorder, at age forty-five. Of note, she had a family history of arthritis; her grandmother had had rheumatoid arthritis and her mother osteoarthritis.

Rheumatoid arthritis is a tough disease—approximately one-third of people stop work within two years of onset and this only increases thereafter. It's also two to four times more common in women than men and, in terms of potential causes, the UK National Health Service (NHS) suggests genetics may play a part, as may hormones and smoking.[1] The National Institute for Healthcare and Excellence Report on RA[2] recommends that those who are newly diagnosed with active RA be on medication within three months.

Aware of the potential side effects of common RA medications, Liz was reticent to go down the conventional route without first exploring other options. Ultimately, she chose to work with a homeopath and from the time of her diagnosis, Liz had done well using a combination of homeopathy and other holistic approaches to support her pain, joint inflammation, sleep, energy levels and mental and emotional wellness.

As laid out in a letter from her rheumatologist to her GP, Liz had a stressful year in 2013-2014 with the deaths of her mother and two of her cats, as well as a bad viral illness for which she was bed-bound for a week. Even so, after consulting with her rheumatologist, she opted to continue supporting her health with nutrition, supplements, homeopathy and other CAM modalities rather than with conventional RA medications, and did so for another nine years, despite dealing with some major life stresses along the way. This was a far cry from the NHS recommendation of three months from diagnosis to drugs.

Liz came to me in 2011 when the homeopath she'd been working with for eleven years retired. Although her RA symptoms were mostly well-managed, they could suddenly flare up. Over time, we would help manage the flare-ups, which were typically triggered by stress.

Liz's symptoms began when she was having challenges in her relationship with her ex-husband—a very stressful point in her life. She was a massage therapist and reflexologist (and would go on to be a brilliant Bowen Therapist too) alongside her job as a nurse. She was, and is, a keen cyclist with a quick sense of humour and often has a cheeky sparkle in her eye. Looking back at her old case notes, a picture emerged of a lot of suppressed emotions, along with a desire to make things right for everyone around her. Liz wasn't always able to articulate what she needed for herself, instead walking the route to make everything okay for everyone else. It made sense to me that she had done well over the years on various potencies of the homeopathic medicine Carcinosin.

Over the next twelve years, we worked with a variety of different homeopathic medicines, including the Carcinosin, as different challenges, such as shingles for example, arose. For twenty-three years, Liz had done well enough managing her RA symptoms overall to forego the conventional medicines typically prescribed for the disease, which is truly amazing! In 2023, Liz decided that it was the right time for her to introduce conventional medication to the complementary medicines she'd been using until then. I'm incredibly grateful to be on Liz's team to support her in doing what feels right for her. Of her experiences with homeopathy during this time, she said:

"Homeopathy has served me well with treating and stabilising both acute and chronic situations. It has helped me deal with personal events, such as divorce, with all that that entails, and

bereavements. The latest amazing treatment was for shingles; the remedies quickly dealt with the symptoms and made my recovery easier without the side effects of antivirals. People have often scoffed when I say it's my 'go to' but I know that I'm in good physical shape and active today because I've chosen to use homeopathy and other alternative therapies."

DIANE

I first met Diane in 2012 on our way to a festival where we were to camp as part of a bigger group that included mutual friends. Standing in a supermarket car park in the July sunshine, we got chatting. 'What do you do?' she asked. 'I'm a homeopath,' I replied. 'Ah,' she said, 'we're not going to get on. I work for AstraZeneca.' Her prediction was incorrect; we got on very well, leaving work aside to have a lovely festival experience, so much so that we kept in touch afterwards.

We didn't discuss our different work backgrounds over the following years, so I admit to being somewhat surprised when one day I received an email from Diane asking if I could recommend a homeopath close to where she lived. In our subsequent conversation, she mentioned that, while open to exploring homeopathy now, if I'd have gone on about it when we first met, she wouldn't have considered it. It was a great reminder of why I've learned to embrace 'minimum dose chatting' around this topic over the years; the laws of homeopathy tend to relate to more than just ailments in the wider world, perhaps including the concept of 'less is more' when offering help and advice.

Fast forward a few years and I know Diane is brilliant at using Nux vomica for helping with hangovers and Arnica for bruising. She also readily shares homeopathic medicines with others to help with minor ailments, having one of the Helios first aid kits.

Recently, Diane had knee surgery and I asked how she was getting on. She replied, 'I'm largely pain-free, thankfully, and improving every week. I'm increasing the distance I can walk but I still walk slowly. For some reason the signal to move my leg takes a while to get from my brain, but the physio says that's normal.' I suggested she might try Hypericum in a low dose to take daily. Hypericum can be a wonderful homeopathic medicine to support our nerves and is often the first medicine to think of if we have an injury causing nerve pain, for example, falling on your coccyx, trapping fingers in a door or similar. Diane started taking the remedy and three weeks later, I had a message from her:

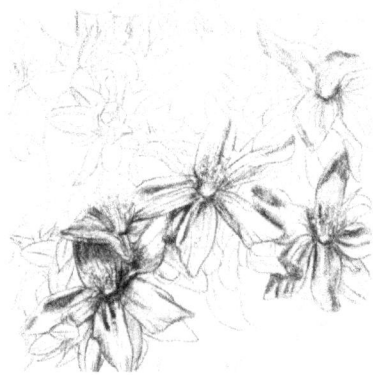

Hypericum

"Thought I'd let you know my issues with delayed messages getting to my legs appear to have resolved. I can now walk pretty much without thinking, and although still walking slightly slower than before, I think this is more to do with my fitness than anything else. So thank you for the remedy. We'll never know whether it did work but coincidentally, my issue resolved. As you know, I do believe there is a place for homeopathy and this has definitely been one of them (along with Nux vom, my go to when I overindulge!). Thanks Em x"

A few months later, Diane got in touch after I'd mentioned I was writing this book and had this to say:

"Hi Em—Well done you writing a book! Thought I'd give you an update on my (knee) progress. I don't know whether the homeopathic remedy worked or not, however I am much recovered and did so pretty quickly after starting it. I certainly think it helped in my recovery. I can now walk at a 'normal' pace and find walking quite straightforward. I'm still getting a little pain if I bend my

knees too much but this is also easing. All things considered, my recovery has been pretty good and definitely faster than many, and I think the homeopathic remedy has helped me on my way (and you can quote me on it!). Diane"

I'm delighted that Diane was open to exploring homeopathy. I'm also thankful that she shared her perspective of how, had our initial conversation upon first meeting gone differently, she might never have sought it out. When I asked her later why she ended up considering homeopathy, she said she'd seen high placebo responses in some clinical trials for conventional medicine and started to realise that there is more involved than just the chemistry that we currently understand. She went on to say that our friendship also played a part: 'As a friend I trusted you to tell the truth. You had credibility with me. Why wouldn't I, with a scientific background, be interested in learning by hearing about the experiences of others? Now, I wouldn't be without some of my remedies!'

7

MENTAL HEALTH

It feels to me that we're currently in a pandemic of mental health challenges. Anxiety and depression make a huge impact on so many lives, and children nowadays are the most medicated they've ever been. An article published in *Psychology Today* in 2021 suggests that in the USA, one in twelve children are on psychiatric drugs, including 1.2 percent of pre-schoolers and 12.9 percent of twelve to seventeen-year-olds,[1] and more than six million children under the age of seventeen are taking some form of psychiatric medication.[2] On my side of the pond, by 2018 the number of antidepressants prescribed to under eighteens in the UK had already surpassed a third of a million, with the fastest growth seen among children under twelve years old. Overall in the UK, there were eighty-six million antidepressant medications prescribed in 2022 and 2023 to an estimated 8.6 million identified patients, whilst prescribing of Central Nervous System (CNS) stimulants and drugs for attention deficit hyperactivity disorder (ADHD) increased by thirty-two percent in adults over eighteen and twelve percent in children seventeen and under.[3]

My daughter, Isla, who is seventeen at the time this book goes to print, has had plenty of talks in school about mental health but not so many about what we may do to help ourselves improve it. Isla thinks there should be therapists in schools providing regular sessions, should children choose to take them, and I, of course, think there should be a homeopath there too! Getting outside in nature, eating well, good sleep and less phone-gazing don't seem to be mentioned much, though they can all make a big difference to our health and well-being. Of course, sometimes medications are needed (and can be lifesaving) but sometimes, they cause unpleasant side effects and people can find taking them difficult. I often wish we had more open discussions on all of the things out there that can help support us through difficult times.

In this section, I'll share the cases of Sarah, who turned to homeopathy after taking antidepressants for years and becoming uncomfortable with the idea of using increasingly more medication to manage her daily life, plus some of the children I've worked with: Nora, Ralf and Ben. However, we'll begin with Jo, who came to homeopathy *before* exploring other options.

Jo

I first met Jo in 2015, when she was in her mid-thirties. She described some physical symptoms that appeared about four months prior—her hair was 'like straw', her nails had been splitting for weeks and she'd put on weight, though she wasn't eating more than usual. She also recognised she was drinking more than was good for her in order to cope with chronic stress. To her credit, as soon as she realised this, she'd almost immediately reduced her alcohol intake to one instead of four bottles of wine a week, begun coating her hair in coconut oil and made some dietary changes.

While Jo felt she was taking care of the physical side of things, she explained how, emotionally, she wasn't where she wanted to be. In general, she told me, she's a really happy person but now felt like a swan, looking serene to everyone around her while furiously paddling away under the surface and feeling like she was at tipping point.

In talking about her personal life, Jo told me that her hopes and dreams for the future were very different than those of her husband. She had previously travelled and lived in Australia, where she felt rested and energised, but in Wales, where she now lived with her family, she was constantly exhausted, even though she was sleeping seven to eight hours each night. She really missed Australia and had this feeling of being 'lost between two sides of the world.' She went on to confide, 'A few years ago, I would have thought being called the perfect wife was the greatest compliment.' Now, she said that role felt restricting. In fact, perfection had been a theme in her life for a long time; she recalled being aware, at age fifteen, that she had to do everything right in order to avoid criticism. It had taken her ages, she said, 'to realise I don't have to be perfect.'

Jo had always been ambitious and wanted to change the world from a young age; she even dreamt at age eleven of being the first woman president of the U.S. She loved nature—watching the stars, spending time in her garden—and needed 'a massive land mass to spread out in.' Being an engaged, aware mother to her son was particularly important to her; she was home-educating him and loved it. However, she'd also become overwhelmed at the demands people placed on her day to day and, though she no longer felt she had the energy, she still found herself frequently helping others. Normally, when in a good place, she told me she was 'light and shiny and had so much energy' but now described herself generally feeling 'dull, quashed and squeezed into a box.'

I reviewed the symptoms relating to Jo and who she was, and was most intrigued by the homeopathic medicine from the fallow deer, Dama dama (which you'll recall I prescribed for Claire in the Respiratory Issues section). This medicine matched Jo's sense of feeling trapped, restricted and stuck, while also having a strong desire to please—and not upset—the group. I gave the Dama dama in a high potency, as a split dose, one to be taken the first night and one the second.

I never had a follow-up session with Jo. We'd initially had an in-person consultation while she was visiting the area and at the time I wasn't doing many online consultations, so we decided she would get in touch if she needed to. We were friends on social media and I'd see occasional updates from her. Later, I would see her posts from both Wales and Australia, where she was looking happy and full of light, but it wasn't until I mentioned in one of my newsletters that I was writing this book that she offered for me to share her story here and she gave a fuller update:

"Hi Em,

That's fantastic you are writing a book! You might remember that you helped me way back in 2015, when I was suffering a real crisis in feeling trapped in my life and responsibilities/people-pleasing roles and it was showing up in my health in a bad way. I have never forgotten your amazing help and my wonderful remedy which was based on a red deer I think. [It was fallow deer but close!]

Happy to report that it took time but I do now have a blended life of travel in Wales and Australia and a sense of security which truly feels in alignment with my son and me. We have a continual focus on our holistic health as a priority, which is a huge and positive shift from where things were in 2015. We are still a family that turns to whole food remedies, and then homeopathy and other energetic remedies, as a first port of call to sustained health and vitality. A lot of that is down to you, Em! Thank you so much!

Warmly,
Jo"

SARAH

Sarah and I met in June 2017 when she was forty-four. Her main reasons for coming to see me were depression and anxiety, which she had experienced for many years. Her depression had started in her teens, but the first time she received treatment for it was when she was in her early twenties. She had essentially been on and off antidepressants since then.

Sarah also had migraine headaches. Her experience of the migraine was feeling dizzy and sick with a throbbing head, usually in her temples or the right frontal area. When her headaches came on, she couldn't bear noise or light, and would have to go to bed, typically sleeping for two to three hours. This would take the worst of it away but she would be left with a 'migraine hangover' (similar to a hangover after drinking alcohol) for two to three days afterwards.

She reported having a ratio of seventy per cent bad days to thirty good. There were blocks of time where she felt okay, which would inevitably be followed by a block of time where she was 'spiralling'. For Sarah, this meant having no energy or motivation and a strong feeling of wanting to hide, to be invisible, to be anonymous or run away from everything in her life. She revealed a fantasy in which she'd run away, pick up casual work somewhere and not stay in any one place for too long, allowing her to be on her own, free from constraint. Even during her better times, her energy was 'never great'. She didn't know if this was due to a physical or emotional condition but noted her energy was somewhat better since she'd stopped eating gluten.

At work, she felt responsible for everything and had to be perfect—she could never be ill and had to have 'an impenetrable exterior'. 'I'm not going to let stuff get to me, not going to show it. I carry all this stuff and no one would ever know. I don't get angry and you'll never see me other than this kind of calm, robotic, emotionless state even if I'm angry or upset.' Sarah described how, if someone on her team was ill, she'd send them home but if it was her, she'd try to think of herself as a robot and just push through.

Going back to her constrained feeling, I asked her what constraint felt like. She replied, 'Like people demanding stuff from me. I can't breathe. I'm responsible for everything. I'm scared of getting it wrong. I don't want to make the decision. I feel panicked and can properly spiral into catastrophe.' Whilst her self-esteem was better than it used to be, she told me that if she did something perfectly, she'd only feel it was equal to everyone else's 'good enough' because she was starting from 'way down here'. In addition, she had fears of heights, travelling at speed, being underground, dark spaces and caves. She also had frequent dreams with themes such as not quite getting somewhere, not quite finishing something or having obstacles that throw whatever she's doing off course.

Her GP had her on a prescription of forty milligrams of Citalopram daily for the depression and on a more recent visit, suggested she add beta blockers to her regimen to help manage her anxiety. Sarah, however, was reluctant to take more medication 'just to manage my day-to-day life'. She had an understanding that her migraines, depression and anxiety were all connected. Our ailments *are* often interconnected but not all of us have Sarah's level of awareness. For Sarah, this recognition dovetailed nicely with the primary homeopathic philosophy that has us looking at people as whole beings, not just separate symptoms.

Based on Sarah's desire to withdraw from everything and to always want to 'get it right', plus her description of an 'impenetrable boundary' around her, combined with her depression, anxiety, low energy levels and low self-esteem along with other symptoms she'd described, I suggested the homeopathic medicine Calcium carbonicum (which, you may recall, helped Ann with her migraines) in a medium potency to be taken daily. The changes within a short space of time were profound.

When we met after a month, Sarah reported that her migraines had stopped and the acute anxiety had gone, allowing her to come off the beta blockers within a few days. In our first consultation, Sarah had rated her migraines (which she'd had for over five years), anxiety and overall well-being all at a four out of six (six being as bad as it could be). Just four weeks later, her assessment scores looked very different. She now rated her migraines at zero, her anxiety at one and her well-being at two. She added a rating for her depression, which she scored at a four. Two months into working together, however, her scores had reduced to migraine zero, anxiety one (except for at bedtime when it tended to increase), depression one and a half and overall well-being two. A further month in, her anxiety was 0.1, depression zero and well-being under 0.5. Over time, and in consultation with her GP, Sarah came off her antidepressants as well. She remains off both medications to this day.

I'm keen to highlight in this book, as I do with my clients, that change isn't always instantaneous. If we've spent years being unwell, it can take time to get to a better place of physical, mental or emotional health. And sometimes, as things change, we need to revisit and refine what we're

Calcarea carbonica

doing. Of note in Sarah's case, the Calc carb stopped helping her after a while and there was a period of time when, despite lots of work, I just didn't feel like I was getting to the right remedy for her. With persistence on both our sides, the penny finally dropped for me and I found a nicely matching medicine which has supported her well.

I'll share Sarah's own reflections a year or so into working with her:

"We worked through and found a remedy. Within a few days, I was able to stop taking the beta blockers, and the associated migraines I'd had were gone. Within two or three months, I expe-

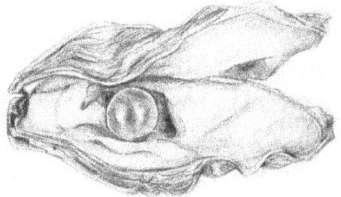

rienced something that I'd never experienced in my life before—a real sense of contentment and inner resilience and a real sense that the world was okay, that I had the skills to deal with it, and that things had stopped fazing me."

Nora

I first met Nora when she was just under two years old. In our consultation, her mum reported she wasn't sleeping as well as she could. She also tended to get more colds than her older sister used to at her age. Nora's mum was looking for homeopathy to generally support Nora's sleep and immune system.

I saw Nora several times over the next couple of years and, while the homeopathic medicines I suggested helped a bit, they didn't offer the impressive change that we saw when we met more recently. Nora, now nine, had by this time developed quite a few tics and some obsessive compulsive disorder (OCD) behaviours, according to her mum. Her family was very accepting of 'her OCDs', but Nora herself said she wished some of them would stop. As is typical with OCD, she couldn't keep from doing them. The particular ritual that frustrated her the most was when she went to bed—she needed the blanket in just the right position, she slept with the exact same ten toys and they had to be 'in the right order' or otherwise 'there'd be chaos'.

In general, Nora was very affectionate and cuddly with her parents, giving lots of kisses when she wanted to. Interestingly, sometimes she would lick them on their arms, asking first if that would be okay. She was very independent but didn't like to be by herself. Her mum said, 'She likes to be left alone but also wants to be around us.' If things didn't go her way, she could get very stressed and think something dreadful could happen, and if something was 'not right' it could be a big issue and would take a long time for Nora to 'level out again'. She hated it when she thought people were cross or frustrated. Cats were important to her; they were her favourite animal and she'd even had a 'creepy dream' the night before we met about a collection of feral cats. She would make beds out of tissue boxes for her soft toys and at mealtimes she'd often feed all her toys as well as herself. Like many kids, her favourite food in the world was ice cream. She also loved to climb.

When it came to matching a remedy for Nora, I didn't want to get caught up in thinking too simplistically. It might have been easy to say, 'Ah, that sounds like a cat remedy would help as cats are something she's talking about a lot.' However, it was also important not to ignore all of the other clues she gave me. So after time considering her case, I had a strong feeling that the medicine Lac felinum (cat's milk, which helped Laura with her dermatitis, as described in the Skin Complaints section) in a high potency might help.

We may often be drawn to our 'remedy archetypes' and it's worth paying attention to what we are attracted to and intrigued by—whether that be in the books we read, the films we love, the stories we write or the games we play. Nora definitely loved anything featuring cats, but she also seemed to fit the picture of this remedy well overall. She was caring, affectionate and particular, and had this interesting blend of being independent and also wanting people around her. I noted that she wanted to make beds for her soft toys and feed them all at the dinner table, which also led me to think a Lac (milk) remedy could be supportive for her.

We met six weeks later for a follow-up session. Nora and her mum both told me Nora had been a lot less stressed out in general and that, after the two-week repeat of the remedy, Nora had had a brief intensification of some symptoms. This, as discussed earlier, can be a good sign that the remedy is a match. Sure enough, Nora's mum now reported she seemed happier, less stressed out and anxious, and more playful, even spending more time outside. There was much less compulsive checking of her toys and stuffed animals at night-time too. In addition, the family had been away for the week and had another trip planned, and Nora wasn't stressed about it at all. Even Nora herself confirmed that her OCD was 'sort of going'.

As Nora's family had used homeopathy for years and was happy with how things were going, we didn't plan for another session but rather for them to get in touch as and when needed. At the time of writing, I enquired if it would be okay for me to share Nora's story and whether they wanted to add anything. Nora's mum replied:

> *"Homeopathy has helped both my kids at various stages in their young lives. I've noticed a big improvement with Nora in particular. As Em said, her anxiety and tics have massively reduced. It's so nice to have a trusted homeopath who knows a fair bit about us to help when needed. Super grateful that I was introduced to homeopathy when my first was a baby."*

RALF

Ralf was two and a half when his mum brought him to see me with sleep issues. He hadn't slept well since birth and was now often restless at night. His dad described him as moving 'like a drill bit—he spins all night.' His most unsettled time was between midnight and four a.m. Most nights, his dad would sleep with him for a while (Ralf wanted to snuggle in close) but did so at the risk of being battered and bruised come morning. All through the night, Ralf kicked, thrashed and spun around in bed. He also didn't nap, though his mum felt he needed to, saying he'd be overtired by the time he went to bed. Further, he sweated a lot at night (in particular on his head) and could then wake feeling cold and clammy.

His mum said of his earlier years, 'He wasn't a settled baby. He had tummy problems and reflux and he never stopped screaming—he screamed and screamed.' Now, in addition to his sleep issues, noises worried him and his mum described how he was 'scared of everything', mentioning things like alarm sensors, the smoke alarm, the kettle, the light on a phone and the train barriers when the lights flashed. Also, while he tended to play independently while someone else was in the room with him, he would get upset if they left.

Because very young children can't tell you much about how they experience their symptoms, as homeopaths much of the treatment choice is based on observation and what we're told by the parents. So, taking into account his sweaty head, fearful nature, restless sleep and the particular time each night that sleep was worse, I decided that I'd give him Calcium carbonicum in a medium potency. You may have noted that this medicine has been mentioned in a few cases—it's one of our 'polychrests' (or commonly-used homeopathic medicines) and has a wide scope of potential uses.

We met again three weeks later and Ralf's mum described how they'd seen a definite change. While he still wanted to sleep with someone, he didn't spin and rotate as much. Though he still tended to be scared about certain things, he was a bit calmer around them. Where before he was nervous about walking down the hall, for example, and would need someone to go with him, now he was going into the hall alone and could even happily play there by himself.

We next met a month later. I then changed the potency of the remedy slightly, and switched to a daily dose, as there were good improvements on the day of the remedy but they seemed to wear off quickly. This did the trick. At our next meeting, his mum described the results as 'amazing'. She told me how he'd even slept through some nights without incident. 'He's so much more settled, it's absolutely unbelievable. Sometimes he still wakes but he just rolls over and goes back to sleep.' Ralf continued with the remedy as needed, increasing potency if it seemed to no longer be helping and, while sleep was never 'perfect', it remained a whole lot better.

As Ralf grew up, the family wondered whether he was displaying traits of being on the autism spectrum. He could be quite aggressive with children his own age and would play alongside—but not cooperate with—others. He tended to get overwhelmed easily and could behave unpredictably at times. Also, he had returned to not wanting to be left alone or move about the house by himself, asking for 'protection' from his siblings. Even going to the toilet by himself was a challenge.

Initially, I thought I'd found a well-matching remedy for Ralf, but there was no response. It took a few attempts before we had a good match. As every homeopath learns—and I've mentioned earlier—a medicine can look great on paper but it isn't always right. And as I've also mentioned, the proof is in the pudding; you'll know it's a good match when you see it and the patient feels it. With Ralf, after a few different homeopathic medicines were tried, our persistence paid off and, after the latest remedy, I received these messages from his mum:

"This week so far, Ralf has used the toilet independently, gone upstairs to his room on his own to get things, and come to think of it, I haven't heard him ask for protection for a while. Also, his class teacher reported to me that he's been interacting with a girl in his class and he told his teacher that he has two friends. This is so amazing and wonderful. I can't thank you enough for helping him!

...and latest update, he played hide and seek at school with four others yesterday and he's tried some new foods too."

It's not always straightforward but when you're able to see changes like this for someone in an uncomfortable state, it's so worth it.

BEN

Ben was four years old when I met with him and his mum in late 2013. His mum described him as a very sensitive and empathic child. For example, he would pick up when his mum wasn't sleeping well, and it would upset him when he saw other parents shouting at their children. He also hated to have people in his space. He was very particular about textures—he didn't like slimy, slippery things like mud or a runny nose, instead preferring dry things like sand and cotton wool. On the whole, he was more introverted and tended to be serious but would also have bursts of laughter and enjoyed a Monty Python-type sense of humour. Ben was often cautious and could be wary of things but also had a seeking, searching nature and could be quite creative. When doing art, like painting, his mum noticed he was very precise and didn't like to get messy. He was also somewhat sensitive to noise, for example, shouting or noisy children and, when hand dryers in public toilets were blowing he would hold his hands over his ears.

Ben's mum had been looking around for the right nursery for him, aware that he was generally good with adults and would play well one to one and in small groups but bigger groups could be much trickier for him. She knew he wouldn't be happy in a large classroom with thirty children in it.

I had also seen Ben when he was younger. At the time, he was very anxious while teething, was particularly sensitive to pain and his sleep wasn't great. He was also very aware of small details and could be clingy to his mum. From seven potentially well-matching homeopathic medicines, I'd selected Calcium carbonicum and afterwards, his mum had seen some improvements. She described how it took the edge off his 'miserableness' and he seemed to have a big leap in development after the remedy.

While Ben had some positive response to the Calc carb back then, I didn't feel the remedy had helped enough for me to suggest it again, so this time I looked for a closer match. It felt to me like there was something deeper, something more to Ben than what this initial medicine was matching. I was aware that his more introverted, seeking, searching temperament fit with the Lanthanide group of remedies and, for him in particular, Lanthanum felt a good match. And, since Ben had had some earlier success with the Calc carb—and I could see aspects relating to the carbon element still in his case—it made sense to suggest Lanthanum carbonicum, which I gave in a high potency.

I didn't meet with Ben and his mum again until March 2015—around a year and a half after our first meeting—when we gathered to discuss a slight skin condition he had developed. His mum said that taking the Lanth carb was the beginning of a big change for him. For example, Ben and his mum had spent time in Australia recently, which he had enjoyed. At the park near their flat, he would now go up to people and say, 'Hi, I'm Ben, do you want to play with me?' This was such a big change from the boy that once typically hid behind his mum on meeting someone new. He was still not 'super brilliant' with crowds of people but if given advance warning, he coped much better with noisy spaces. While he was still sensitive, this side of him felt more in balance and held him back less. He was much better at trying new things and was overall 'much more adventurous in all ways'. His parents had chosen to home-educate him and he was thriving in that environment and, in general, doing really well. Given that the Lanth carb had been so beneficial for Ben in so many areas, we repeated it, after which his skin condition cleared up.

When Ben's mum read through his story prior to sharing it here, she wrote:

"Oh my goodness, I got quite teary reading those (old) case notes as they were just SO accurate and you had recorded so well my descriptions of how things were and how Ben in particular felt. It really took me right back and reminded me of just how hard and intense it was when Ben was out of balance at four, and just how much of a difference your support as a skilled homeopath made!

Ben, at fourteen, is still thriving. He's definitely always going to be an introvert and a highly sensitive person but he's happy and very confident and he knows his own energy levels and boundaries. He goes to an online high school now, as well as to a circus school

(I would never have imagined that!) and he's in regular contact with his friends all over the world."

I really love how a well-matching homeopathic medicine can have such wide-ranging effects, not only in alleviating physical complaints but also in helping someone simply feel more comfortable in the world.

8

Multiple Issues

You may by now have noticed that quite a few of the clients' stories highlighted in this book were dealing with health issues aside from those presented in that particular section. For example, Claire in the Respiratory Issues section also had work-related stress; Juliet in the Skin Complaints section was experiencing stress due to family loss and Sarah in the Mental Health section had migraines alongside her anxiety and depression. As homeopaths, we often see people who are experiencing a variety of symptoms which may initially appear unrelated; however, the mind, body and spirit are intimately connected and so we often see a constellation of issues that may all improve or resolve when we approach health holistically, as homeopathy does.

This is so often true that, in fact, I struggled with the idea of separating the stories into sections based on one primary set of symptoms. While it does give the book a logical structure—presenting an insight into how homeopathy might help with a particular kind of issue—it is unusual for someone to come to me with a single complaint. The following three stories detail my work with clients who sought me out with a more complex array of symptoms.

Anne

When we met in December 2022, Anne came to me with a variety of issues including hair loss with an itchy scalp; red and sore toe tips; a heavy, congested feeling in her legs, ankles and feet; and gastrointestinal inflammation with loose stools/diarrhoea.

She was also struggling with herpes-like symptoms. She described them as mildly inflamed, raised areas which shifted about and were accompanied by a unique nerve sensation. She had had similar lesions in the past, which had cropped up sporadically, and she was aware that they were triggered by stress and eating too many nuts. However, she'd never seen them quite like this before. She described a particular area at the base of her spine which looked like 'a red/brown leech' with a scab-like quality. It was longer-lasting than usual, with the same nerve sensation.

She felt that all of these issues were connected to the bout of Covid she'd experienced in July of that same year. She told me that for her, Covid had been really bad. She had used homeopathic medicines to help get through the acute stages of it and had seen an acupuncturist post-Covid, as she felt she needed more support.

Even though her toes were pretty painful, she said it was her hair loss that was driving her crazy. She described how she would find piles of hair everywhere—on the floor, on the table, on the pillow. As far as the heaviness in her legs went, she said it always felt better to be constantly moving; she really hated standing still.

Aside from her physical symptoms, we talked about her general nature—her likes, dislikes, fears and challenges—as well as where she felt most comfortable in the world. She spoke about working a small farm, the way she liked to be alone, the fact that she often felt like she was in fight or flight mode, and lots more.

I decided to give her Sepia, indicated by her desire to be in motion (and feeling better for it) and her feeling of fight or flight, as well as her physical symptoms, all of which fitted this medicine too. I suggested a medium potency, as a split dose, to be repeated in two weeks if there had been no change.

As a side note, Anne, who had a lot of knowledge about homeopathy, having worked with it herself, told me she was baffled at first by why I'd given her this particular remedy. Sepia is often thought of in the older texts as a 'worn out washer woman' remedy—very much a woman's medicine with symptoms related to hormonal changes (although ironically, the first prover of the medicine was actually a man). Often the books, particularly older texts, seem to focus a little more on a medicine's match to the more negative state, so I'm grateful to the teachers who also shared the positive aspects of the medicine picture with me. Interestingly, I had suggested Sepia for Anne before she shared that her mum had taken weekly hormone injections prior to getting pregnant with her. Had I known this earlier, it could have given me an inkling that a homeopathic medicine with a strong link to hormones could be helpful, but we were still onto a good thing, even without that awareness.

We met a month later and she updated me on her progress. After taking the Sepia that first night, she said she'd slept great. Then her symptoms intensified over the next three to four days, which Anne thought to be a potential aggravation due to the remedy, so she stayed the course. After that, she told me she'd had some huge positive changes and since then, she'd felt really good.

Given her response, we decided to repeat the dose after two weeks due to a small relapse in her symptoms, and she continued to see positive progress. Her herpetic eruptions had reduced, the night sweats had gone and not returned, and her gastrointestinal problems had improved. She had previously rated them at seven or eight out of ten in terms of severity (with ten being worst) and now saw them as four or five out of ten. She thought her hair loss had reduced a little, though it was still going on. Her toe pain (also referred to as 'Covid toes'[1]) was better but hadn't fully resolved and the congestion in her legs had decreased some, especially in the first few weeks.

The fight or flight feeling she had been experiencing had improved tremendously. In addition, she'd seen her acupuncturist the week after she'd taken the first dose, who said her pulses had never been so good. Since they had worked together for eight years, the acupuncturist knew Anne fairly well and was surprised at the result and, with no other explainable reason than the Sepia, they were both happy with it. Finally, though Anne was now struggling with some financial issues, she said she was handling it better than she thought she would and attributed that to the remedy.

We're never going to stop life happening but if we can bring in supportive elements that help us experience things with more ease, well, why wouldn't we? Given all that Anne had going on, if we take a second to reflect upon the changes from just three tablets so far, it's frankly quite brilliant!

Later, Anne's toes began bothering her again pretty badly, so we repeated a dose of Sepia. A step back following improvement may often be a sign that it's time to repeat a remedy. She continued with the Sepia for a time and improvements continued—her digestive symptoms and circulation were better, the hair loss had stopped and her red, painful toes all cleared up.

During one of our follow-up sessions, Anne mentioned she'd been given the remedy Thuja years ago and didn't feel she'd finished working with it. Along with her intuitive feeling about the medicine and her working knowledge of homeopathy, there was easily a case to be made for giving her this remedy with her symptom profile, so I was happy to go along with the suggestion. I definitely don't feel it always has to be me instructing the process. I am open to debate and discussion.

This was what I heard back after she took it: 'All doing well here with Thuja. Nose and eyes seem eased. My spirit felt very good after talking to you.' She saw some improvements for several months and she felt the Thuja helped clear several other symptoms.

We next met in September 2023—nine months after our initial consultation—when Anne was experiencing some very challenging circumstances, particularly around her finances. This was causing her a fair amount of stress and she was experiencing some physical changes, including nose sores, some depression and funny smelling urine. This time, I suggested taking Arsenicum album in a medium high potency.

That same evening I received a short email from her: 'I just took the remedy. Thank you Em. It may be my imagination, but I feel better already.' The following day she sent this email: 'Thank you, Em, for the Arsenicum. I'm so grateful to you—it helped me get my feet back under me and lifted a huge amount of depression. I feel energy this morning to work in the garden and make lists to prepare to go help my sister.' Several days later she reported: 'The Arsenicum has helped me emotionally (Thank you!) and the strange urine smell is hugely improved also. Nose sores improving too.'

To date, Anne's story continues. Hers is a testament to the fact that, not only can homeopathy resolve physical and emotional symptoms, it can help us cope with challenging situations, bringing more ease and joy, which in turn can assist in healing. As life brings us new experiences, this means a return to health isn't always as straightforward as taking one remedy, and sometimes it can take time before we see improvements. We may need to change the medicine. It may take one remedy to help us through something acute and another to help with long-standing issues. Anne's case demonstrates that through a spirit of collaboration, and the open sharing of information, we can see some really positive shifts in health and overall well-being.

GEORGE

George was sixty-six when he first came to me with symptoms he'd had for the last eighteen months, which had started after he'd had an Akashic past life retrieval session. He told me that his most important physical sensation was 'as if someone had beaten me up' and he described how his whole body would hurt, which related to some of the past life experiences he discussed with me.

Furthermore, he was experiencing low vitality, low energy and joint and muscle pain, especially in the mornings. As with many people, he also mentioned other issues—a heart valve disorder (triggered in 2020 after some strenuous activity) and scaly skin/scalp, which he'd had since childhood.

George was very creative; he especially enjoyed working with sound and taking and sharing photographs of the beautiful island where he lived. He considered himself a free spirit; he had travelled and explored the world for work and he also had a sense of curiosity and a desire for spiritual experiences. Unfortunately one of the main effects of his symptoms was that he couldn't be as active as he once was. He did find, however, that the joint and muscle complaints felt better by swimming in the sea, by stretching and after moving. George also mentioned that he was a people-pleaser—he wanted everyone to be happy, he often took on a supportive role for those around him, love was a powerful emotion for him, and being of service was a theme that ran throughout his life. He could be sensitive to surrounding energies and, while this meant he enjoyed connecting with people, it also meant he needed to take time out to be alone and practise grounding to maintain his energy.

I suggested George take the homeopathic medicine Ginseng in a medium potency. Ginseng is another medicine I haven't given before nor since, but was one that matched his symptoms well. Here again is where the wonder of homeopathy's amazing repertories (indexes of symptoms) comes in. I work with the repertory for every case that I see, and often I know of the suggested medicines that come through the search. However, at times

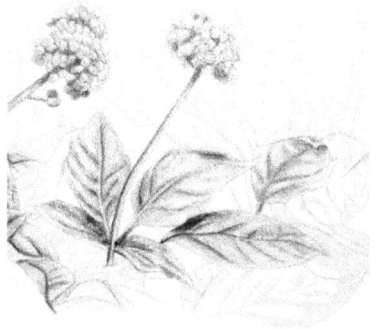

Ginseng

ones will come up that I've not used or even heard of before. If we were to only work with medicines we know, we would be incredibly limited, and using the various repertories at our disposal means we have access to a much wider range of remedies that may help. The repertories, the many *Materia Medica* texts, and information about provings of homeopathic medicines all provide a brilliant system that helps us narrow down our initial selection of potential medicines. In each case I always consult the books after my repertory search to help confirm the final choice.

Not long after our first session George sent me an email to offer his observations after taking the first dose:

> *"1. Less pain in the carpal area (joint) of left hand.*
> *2. Less pain overall in joints.*
> *3. No plugged ears for the first half of the day and no plugged ears the following day.*
> *4. Very restful sleep.*
> *5. Overall feeling of wellness despite the fact that I was out and about in steep terrain in a heatwave.*
> *6. Felt exhausted when I returned home.*
> *7. Muscle stiffness and tightness much reduced.*
> *8. Heart, appetite are well.*
> *9. After an afternoon nap, woke up with the shakes, feeling very cold, hands were freezing. Had to put on a winter robe de chambre and lie down.*
> *10. Above condition lasted for an hour to an hour and a half. Then temperature went back to normal. Ambient temperature felt even warmer than it was.*
> *11. Broke out in scaly skin around the chin area."*

I responded to his email, thanking him for the update and confirming for him that it was an encouraging start: 'It sounds like a really good reaction to the Ginseng and I am tentatively hopeful about progress,' I wrote. Back in the day, as a newly qualified homeopath, I might have been dancing around the room. Now,

I tend to go with a 'tentatively hopeful' and 'let's wait and see' attitude, as life can happen, things can change and time will tell us more.

George and I met for a follow-up session after a month or so and he told me he was really well. Most of his symptoms were improved; the only hint of the muscle and joint pain that he'd previously had all over his body was in his right pelvic area and left arm, and they only bothered him once in a while. His energy seemed to be in a good place, in fact, he'd surprised himself as he recently had a late night out and really enjoyed it. He noticed that while being out with friends previously, he would have needed to go to bed in the midst of it but now he was happy, chatting and having interesting conversations. He also hadn't felt the need to swim, which he was compelled to do previously to help with his pain.

George was content to repeat the remedy if he felt it was needed. As he was familiar with homeopathy, having used it extensively in the past, he didn't feel like he required another session at this stage, opting instead to meet again if things didn't continue to improve. I'm a big fan of empowering people to support their own health and if a client is comfortable repeating a remedy and asking for more support when they feel they need it, I'm all for it.

MAAYAN

Maayan was thirty-five when we first met in 2023. She had heard me talking on a podcast and discussed the possibility of seeing a homeopath with her osteopath, who thought it could be a great idea to have one on her team. She also had a six-month old baby, and consulted me separately for homeopathic support for her baby's dry skin and teething challenges. Maayan told me she was looking for help with eczema, anxiety, stress, headaches and stress-induced irritable bowel syndrome (IBS).

She had been diagnosed with chronic migraines at age nine. Although they were now down to headache level (no longer migraines), she'd noticed an increase in them since giving birth. Also, her sinuses were frequently blocked and she often felt a thick mucus at the back of her throat, which led her to typically have to clear her throat before speaking. Her eczema had initially appeared on her hands and wrists quite severely twelve years ago. She'd managed it with natural products ever since, though it kept cropping up lightly in one place or another. It was currently on her wrist and she wondered if that was because she'd recently rubbed an essential oil on that area. (Of note, she was later able to use the oil without flaring the eczema at all after using homeopathy.) She'd had the anxiety as long as she could remember and was aware that stress made all her symptoms worse. The stress could also trigger severe stomach issues (diarrhoea, IBS) that might last for months, and she also noticed that when she scheduled a time to meet someone or needed to say no to plans with someone, this would particularly cause her stress, often resulting in a headache.

Our initial consultation took place online in June 2023 when Maayan further shared that decision-making exaggerated her symptoms and the last time she'd had a big decision to make, she had a bad flare of IBS which only cleared when she resolved what she was going to do. During our session, she said her IBS symptoms had got worse that week, though she couldn't see any reason for this particular flare-up.

Maayan had seen a doctor for her IBS several years earlier and was told that all was well. In my opinion, IBS, like some other diagnostic labels, is an umbrella term covering lots of symptoms. I think this highlights the importance, as with any ailment, to know how you are experiencing your symptoms. For Maayan, she would feel pressure in her abdomen, a lot of gurgling and an increase in urgency and frequency of needing to use the toilet. On a morning, she'd need to visit the toilet suddenly and on an evening as she was putting her baby to bed, there'd be the same urgency, which might require her to go between three and five times.

Maayan was a keen researcher and, with any decision, she would weigh up all the information she'd gleaned in order to determine the right course of action. Though reaching a conclusion might be difficult and take some time, she would put one hundred percent effort into whatever action she chose to take. Preparation and planning were key aspects of who she was and she did these things well, always striving for perfection. She was also a prolific list maker—she told me she currently had three hundred and sixty-five open tabs on her phone. In addition, routine was key for her in avoiding headaches—changes such as job interviews or time pressures could bring them on. In her job, prior to taking maternity leave, she'd overseen multiple projects requiring much organisation. It was a job that suited her well.

After working on her case, I had a strong feeling that the homeopathic medicine Manganum phosphorus might help support her. I gave this in a high potency, to be taken as a split dose (one the first evening and one on the second evening), repeating in two weeks if she saw no change.

We met again in six weeks and Maayan told me she'd taken the first two pills and not felt the need to take another dose. Prior to taking the remedy, she had also noted a heaviness in her chest but within a couple of days, she experienced a new feeling of lightness in the same area. The eczema on her wrist had cleared up about a week after taking the tablets; previously it had been getting bigger and bigger. Now, she had a small patch of it on her fingers and at the back of her head but that was it. Her sinuses also felt clear.

When I enquired about the headaches and anxiety, she mentioned she'd found a lump in her thyroid but said even with that, she hadn't felt overwhelmed, which in the past she would have done. She'd only had a few headaches in the last six weeks and, though she still experienced anxiety in relation to certain topics, she was no longer getting a headache when leaving the house or trying to get to an appointment. When she first saw me, she rated her anxiety at nine out of ten but now she put it around four. Her stress headaches, which were a nine or ten in terms of intensity, were also now at four. The duration of her headaches had also reduced, down from several hours to perhaps fifteen or twenty minutes. In terms of frequency, they went from three to four per week to a total of one or two over the last six weeks. Maayan had also been more social and had even made some new friends.

On the downside, she reported that her IBS symptoms had been bad and she was also working on them with her osteopath. As a result, she'd made some dietary changes and said that while the symptoms were the same in intensity, they were perhaps not quite as frequent.

Meeting in another six weeks, she was still feeling much calmer, the eczema on her wrist had never returned and her fingers were now clear. While the patch on her head was still present, it had continued to get smaller. She'd only had one headache since we'd last spoken.

Her IBS symptoms were still the main challenge. She described them as taking over her evenings—whilst putting her baby to bed, she'd be going back and forth to the toilet. She'd had another blood test ordered by her doctor and while waiting for the results, I felt the IBS symptoms needed a slightly different tack. This time, I gave the homeopathic medicine Croton tiglium in a medium potency, as a split dose, to be repeated in a week if no change. We also planned to continue with the monthly dose of Mang phos, as it seemed to be supporting everything else well. As I do with other clients, I encouraged Maayan to get in touch with me at any point with questions or concerns before we next met.

Generally, I meet people for follow-up sessions four to six weeks after they've taken their initial remedy. This time interval allows space for the remedy to act. I'm always happy, however, to stay in touch by email in between if people have questions. In fact, I'll tell my clients the one thing I don't like is if someone comes back and says something like, 'I had a question and it was really bugging me, but I didn't want to disturb you, so I thought I'd wait until we met, but I've been really worrying about...' I tell those I'm working with that I would so much rather take a few moments to reply than have someone sit and worry at home. Chances are, I can answer their questions fairly quickly.

We met again in a month, though we'd kept in touch by email to adjust how often she was taking the Croton tiglium. Maayan reported that her IBS symptoms themselves were more or less the same but the frequency had reduced significantly. Now she was only going to the toilet once in the late evening, though when she did go, it was similarly 'explosive'. At this point, she had been referred by her GP for a colonoscopy and rectal examination but, for our part, we continued the remedies and met again a month later.

At this session, Maayan told me she hadn't been to the toilet yet that morning—which she felt great about—and overall, her symptoms were so much better. She rated her improvement in her IBS symptoms at eighty-five to ninety percent. In the meantime, she'd received a formal diagnosis of ulcerative colitis (UC), which the doctors acknowledged could be activated by stress. The colorectal team suggested she have a colonoscopy in six months and also wanted her to take medication for the UC. As Maayan was still breastfeeding, she was reluctant to take the medications, particularly as she currently had no symptoms from the IBS. Happily, her thyroid results had come back fine; her doctor was simply monitoring with a follow-up in one year.

The following month, Maayan told me she no longer felt she needed even the homeopathic remedy for her UC symptoms as there weren't any. She currently rated her IBS/UC symptoms as one hundred percent better. She'd spoken with her GP, who was open-minded about her using homeopathy. The GP offered that, while she couldn't explain why it might be working, she was happy to monitor Maayan and suggested a blood test and stool sample in January. Since her doctor was also a former gastroenterologist, Maayan felt well supported with this plan.

We met in January 2024. Maayan reported that her colitis, eczema and headaches were all still clear, though she had some return of her sinus symptoms and still noticed some remaining anxiety. To date, we continue to work together and, though her symptoms haven't been a quick fix, it's been a real joy to see the progress that she's made so far. It's a real pleasure to work with such an engaged client, as well as a supportive GP.

9

MANAGING SIDE EFFECTS

OF MEDICATIONS AND TREATMENTS

As I've mentioned earlier, I think that conventional medical science is utterly remarkable. Lifesaving. Brilliant. I am grateful to live in a world where it exists. Sometimes, however, there can be side effects that create additional burdens, which homeopathy may help to relieve.

Surgery is a good example—it can take some time to recover from an operation but there are now studies that suggest homeopathic remedies can assist patients with the process. In a Tanzanian study I heard of via colleagues who work there, practitioners in a surgical ward started one group of women post-surgery on the homeopathic remedy Bellis perennis, while the other group recovered as normal. After a few weeks, the medical team decided that it was unethical to continue the study as the group using the Bellis perennis were recovering so much faster and with less pain. So whilst the trial results never saw the light of day (as the study was abandoned), the women and medics saw first-hand the results of using homeopathy alongside surgical interventions.

Written up in the *European Journal of Plastic Surgery*, another study examined the use of Arnica and Bellis perennis post-mastectomy and immediate breast reconstruction. Their findings saw a reduction in the need for opioid pain medication and the risk of seroma post-surgery: 'Arnica Montana and Bellis Perennis have been shown to reduce seroma formation and opioid intake following mastectomy and reconstruction. As this treatment lacks side effects and is inexpensive, it should serve as a valuable treatment adjunct in patients undergoing mastectomy and reconstruction.'[1]

I'm grateful to my dad and my sister, whose brief stories I share in this section about how integrating homeopathy helped each of them manage various side effects of cancer treatment. Both my dad and my sister worked with other practitioners at times, and their stories here are the moments where they reached out for help from me. As I mentioned in my daughter Isla's case (in the Respiratory Issues section), it's often hard to treat family. In both instances I knew that's what my role was—to be family—a supportive daughter and sister respectively whilst they worked with others for support. That said, when they asked for help with issues as they arose, of course I did what I could.

Louise's case, which follows their stories in this section, was the catalyst for this book. I initially wrote it up to share on my blog and just kept writing. I had no grand plan to write a book, but the words flowed and here we are!

This section finishes with the story of Bex, who is happily now doing brilliantly but who had quite a journey to get there.

Roy (My Dad)

My dad, Roy, was diagnosed with prostate cancer. I'd like to add that he was a 'supportive sceptic' of me working with homeopathy for many years. He'd never tell me to my face, nor would he say anything behind my back (he's a bit of a gentleman really), but I'm not convinced that he thought homeopathy was any good.

Early in his conventional medical treatment, he texted me to ask if there was anything I could do to help with a bleeding rectum due to his radiotherapy. While hospital staff were unconcerned—it's a common side effect—it obviously wasn't pleasant to experience. I gave him two homeopathic medicines to take. By the next day, the bleeding had reduced greatly and by the following day, it was all gone. The change to his symptoms was beautiful to hear about.

Some time later, I was out at dinner with him to celebrate him finishing his radiotherapy. I asked him how he was feeling and he replied, 'Good, except when I wee it's like passing hot needles.' I suggested that the homeopathic medicine Cantharis may help with his burning urination, which he took once when he got home, then again later that evening. His symptoms disappeared. No more peeing needles. It started to creep back a bit the next morning, so I suggested one repeat dose, then to repeat as needed if the symptoms returned. While my dad may have been a sceptic before, he's totally on board now and had been for quite some time prior to his recent experiences detailed here. He and I have talked about the fact that it's understandable that some people don't 'get' homeopathy. In so many ways it makes no sense, at least in terms of our current model of scientific enquiry, except perhaps at the cutting edges. Still, when you take it and it works, it becomes quite simple. Dad said to me once, 'When you get it right, it's like magic.'

There are many areas where I believe the integration of complementary and alternative medicines (CAM) with conventional treatments can be beneficial to patients, and assisting with the side effects of cancer treatments is just one of them.

Ruth (My Sister)

My sister Ruth found out in 2016, at the age of thirty-five, that she had a large, malignant brain tumour. My sister is probably one of the most determined people out there. Once she's set her mind to something, she's able to single-mindedly follow that track. And healing from this was a mission she was on. Ruth had surgery, radiotherapy and chemotherapy and she used many CAM approaches, including homeopathy, alongside these interventions. She was told that there still remained about two cubic centimetres of tumour that the surgery was unable to remove. While early scans showed no noticeable change, for the last six years they have shown no evidence of disease. There is no longer any measurable tumour, despite the fact that, at the time of diagnosis, Ruth was told (in no uncertain terms) that the radiotherapy and chemotherapy would not shrink the tumour, it would only hopefully stop it from growing. Now, her consultants say that the chemotherapy and radiotherapy must have shrunk it, even though they told her definitively that this wouldn't happen.

Ruth used many approaches, so of course we can't say which was the most helpful in terms of supporting the tumour shrinking and her overall health, and she doesn't mind this at all. During her treatment and beyond, homeopathic remedies helped her with post-operative constipation and lots more. Arsenicum album, Nux vomica and others helped her cope with nausea and sickness from the chemotherapy medications, whilst other homeopathic medicines helped with burning sensations during radiotherapy. Hypericum perforatum helped to significantly decrease her neuropathy pain following chemotherapy. Neuropathy post or during chemotherapy is something I've frequently seen resolve relatively quickly, even in cases where the client was told they may have to stop the chemotherapy if the neuropathy didn't clear up.

It's wonderful to be able to walk alongside someone in support of their treatment choices, whatever that may look like to the individual you're working with.

Louise

Louise and I had chatted on the phone before she made her first appointment. Aged forty-one, she told me that she'd been a well, happy, busy mum prior to having a Covid vaccine booster, to which she'd had a bad reaction. I know this can be a difficult topic to discuss and I'm not interested in entering into a debate on the issue. I am aware that this coronavirus has been challenging for many. I am also aware that, at times, the effects from preventative measures can be challenging too[2] and this is the case with Louise and the side effects she experienced.

Louise described the situation as follows: 'In November 2021, I had the Covid vaccine booster. Within three hours, I started to have stroke-like symptoms. My gait changed, I was unable to pick up my left leg (I had to drag it) and my right leg was turned in. Eventually I used walking backwards and grounding, which helped, but my legs can often stop working. I have absence episodes, brain fog, tics and what appear to be functional seizures. I have pain and sensations in my arms and legs, struggle hugely to travel and can feel really funny-headed, not dizzy but not well.'

Louise had tried a wide range of therapies and approaches, many of which had helped her, however, her symptoms were still significant and debilitating. She told me, 'These are the things I have tried that seem to have helped: Emotional Freedom Technique (EFT), yoga, meditation, deep heat cream, hot showers, heated bags, lip trills, cold water on my face daily, regulating breathing, hypnotherapy, resetting myself, pacing, managing sensory sensitivities using ear plugs, and being kind to myself and reducing the pressure I place on myself and my expectations.' She had also had a few sessions of physiotherapy and had asked to be referred back.

I asked Louise about the effects the symptoms were having on her life. She wrote, 'I can no longer drive, travelling is really hard, walking is difficult (as is the aftermath from it), so getting out is hard. In fact, pretty much everything is impacted [in terms of my quality of life]. I can't be the mum I was. I feel I have lost myself and also lost my joy. Every aspect of my life has changed. I generally just feel pretty unwell a lot of the time.'

We met online in August 2023 and discussed Louise's current symptoms in more detail, as well as who she was before this happened and lots more. When talking about her life at this time, Louise described how she would 'try to push through'. For example, though travelling was difficult, she did it anyway because she'd 'go insane' if she didn't do anything. This was an even more impressive feat given that for her, motion made everything worse. She said her arms and legs could go heavy, numb and dead and she could have a burning sensation in them too. When I asked her to describe what she meant by 'burning', she said that, when putting her feet down, 'it feels as if they're shattering. It goes right into my hips… it feels as if they're breaking.' She also mentioned that she had been offered a medication for her symptoms but was warned that it could put her into a 'vegetative state'. Due to the severity of her symptoms, she was seriously considering taking it but hadn't so far.

In terms of her personality, Louise described herself as highly sensitive—picking up on subtleties from people and the environment around her—and a perfectionist. She clarified that it wasn't as though she felt in competition with others, it was more about doing things perfectly for herself. She told me she constantly overthinks and that she's 'very strong, determined and stubborn'. She added that when well, she was joyful and playful, adding, 'I'm the one with the big loud laugh.'

I gave her Nux vomica, a medicine commonly used in homeopathy. People fitting the Nux vom picture may have a perfectionist streak and can be high performers—I think of it as a remedy for Wall Street bankers, as that 'work hard, play hard' idea fits well. Louise fitted this picture too, which was evident in the determination she'd shown in trying so many things to help her get back on her feet. When we consider that Nux vom is from the Strychnine tree (full name *Strychnos nux-vomica*), and think about the effects of strychnine toxicity, it's not surprising that there are so many neurological complaints in the picture—tics, twitches and more may be helped by this homeopathic medicine. I gave a low potency to be taken twice, then repeated in two weeks. We corresponded by email over the next few weeks to adjust this as needed.

We met a month later. Louise reported that after taking the first two doses, travelling felt better than it had for the last two years. Then the symptoms worsened again, during which time she tested positive for Covid. It wiped her out energy-wise and made her symptoms worse for a bit but at this session, I was encouraged to hear her say she felt better in general, revealing 'I'm seeing glimmers of myself.'

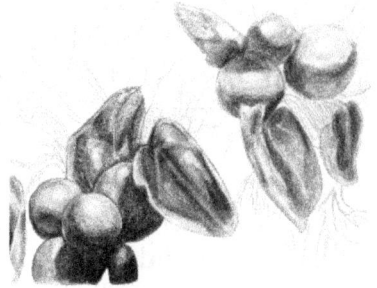

Nux vomica

Before we met, it could take fifty minutes for Louise to get downstairs because her legs wouldn't work, and she might end up with tics or even seizures in the process. Now she said, 'I just walk down the stairs.' Apart from a couple of seizures during the period when she tested positive for Covid, she wasn't having them anymore. She was still having some tics, but while before she rated them eight or nine out of ten, they were now four or five. Overall, she described the feeling of her nervous system calming down, and said that she was more present and playful and had experienced more joy over the last month. She also told me that two weekends ago, she had gone swimming two days in a row. This meant taking two buses each way, which she handled brilliantly. She told me she couldn't have imagined doing that before.

Others had noted changes too—someone close to her told her that after the initial two doses, it was like 'having her back' in that moment. Louise was also aware of a lot of old stress held in her body and was intuitively using yoga, Tension & Trauma Releasing Exercises (TRE®) and other somatic work to support herself.

As we chatted, Louise used a phrase that really resonated with me. She said, 'I finally feel in the here and now.' I have a wonderful teacher, Jeremy Sherr, who talks about exactly that—how a well-matched homeopathic medicine can bring us from the 'there and then' into the 'here and now'. This is based on the idea that many of us spend most of our time in the past or the future, either ruminating on things that have happened or worrying about what's to come. It's not uncommon for those who take a well-matched homeopathic medicine to express feeling more present. It's something I've heard in my practice many times now.

As we ended our meeting, Louise said, 'On reflection, I do feel a lot better. I have hope. Things are different. It's been a hard two years but working with homeopathy has been transformative.'

We met again a month later and her improvements had continued. She'd had one seizure (as a reminder, they were happening almost daily when we first met, if not even more frequent at times) and the tics had reduced to about a quarter of the frequency as before. During this session, I saw little evidence of them, while in our previous sessions I had observed them pretty clearly. She was doing lots more activities and had taken the bus by herself several times (a major achievement). In general, all areas were showing improvement.

Most people clearly do not respond to a vaccine the way Louise did. While there is evidence to support an under-reporting of incidents such as hers,[3] what is more important to me is that there are people suffering, and that homeopathy, as well as other alternative and complementary modalities, may help.

While Louise's progress wasn't always linear—there had been ups and downs—the trend for Louise was solidly in the right direction. I give her a whole heap of credit for using an extensive range of tools to support her recovery and for not giving up. I feel certain that her determination has helped carry her through, along with the Nux vom and other options she's used. I am hopeful she may see a full recovery, grateful that she added homeopathy to her toolkit and thrilled that it has brought her such positive results.

I'd like to share Louise's thoughts on the process:

"Em listened intently, asked questions with curiosity, really heard what I was saying and, from this, suggested the remedy that I've

come to see as magic—a magic that I don't question. I go with it, I accept, appreciate, value and I am grateful for it for it because of what it is—life changing."

In the summer of 2024, Louise had an active family holiday overseas—something she never thought she'd be able to do again.

Bex

I met Bex for the first time in February 2021 when she was seventeen and dealing with chronic fatigue syndrome (CFS).

Bex's health seemed to take a turn for the worse at the age of fifteen, after she'd had the human papillomavirus (HPV) vaccine in January 2019 and then a booster in May of that same year. At the time, with the support of her parents, she had visited multiple doctors and had had several hospital appointments. Her hospital records state that she had unexplained symptoms since the HPV vaccine.

Her pediatrician initially charted her primary symptoms as dizzy spells, nausea and what could potentially be narcolepsy. An electrocardiogram (ECG) was ordered due to abnormal heart activity which suggested that it may no longer be safe for her to continue gymnastics (an activity she'd been involved with for some time), sports and other strenuous activities. This was less than a month after her HPV booster. Further blood tests revealed a diagnosis of POTS[4] and she was referred to a neurologist for the possible narcolepsy.

Bex started getting even more ill in September 2019. She had been away on a summer holiday in Italy and afterwards, had a bout of diarrhoea and sickness 'like never before', followed by a feeling of very low energy. She then started sleeping for longer and longer periods. At the same time, her face had swelled up, particularly her eyelids and lips.

Of note, prior to our initial consultation, she had informed me, among other things, that as a young child she had eczema all over her body, which her mum mentioned had seemed to occur shortly after her childhood vaccines.[5] I want to say here that I am not against vaccines, and whilst health issues post-vaccination may be rare, the Medicines and Healthcare Products Regulatory Agency (MHRA) do inform us that side effects can result from any medication. As a practitioner, I'm not here to have an opinion on this. Should someone seek my thoughts on it, I always refer them to discuss the topic with their GP or healthcare provider. But back to Bex.

Though Bex had been told by medical specialists what may have caused her health challenges, she had been given no idea what to do about them and she was really struggling. We met online in the evening, as that was the time she was most likely to be awake and able to chat to me. That day, like most, she'd been asleep all day. In general, Bex rarely got out of bed, sleeping up to twenty hours, and was awake only to shower and eat (though sometimes if it was a bad day, she was fed in bed). When awake, she was still exhausted and also in pain. She had a lot of muscle and joint pain (fibromyalgia), describing it like period cramp but in her ankles, elbows and legs. She didn't tolerate sunlight well—she didn't like it if her mum opened the curtains nor did she like the light on in rooms. She also found heat annoying. In general, for the last two years she was barely coping and was certainly not living the full life of a teenager. She wasn't in school, she barely saw her friends and if she did, she would then be in bed for the rest of the weekend.

Before this happened, Bex had loved to play sports, having played tennis, netball and badminton, and also enjoyed dance and gym. Referring back to the ECG she'd had, she said, 'I had to stop as my heart rate went too high.' In fact, she preferred sports over academic work and could be quite competitive.

Personality-wise, she could be fun but also get angry easily and tended to be serious and strong-minded. If she was told to do something, it would make her not want to do it but if left on her own, she'd likely get around to doing whatever task was asked of her. She was also shy with people she didn't know well and could suffer from significant anxiety at times. She told me she enjoyed being by the sea doing things like body boarding, surfing, stand-up paddle boarding and kayaking, as well as swimming. When she was little, she'd been scared of the dark (and still was, though she also didn't like bright light). Also of note, she used to have dreams of being kidnapped, which would freak her out, and recounted how she'd almost been kidnapped in reality on two separate occasions, once on her lane and once elsewhere.

I reviewed her case, keeping Bex's personality and symptoms in mind, and decided to give her Stoichactis kenti, a homeopathic medicine made from a sea anemone. This is another example of where the beauty of the repertories shines through. Prior to this case, I had no concept of this homeopathic medicine. In our consultation, I wasn't particularly thinking that I was looking for a remedy from the sea but as I've mentioned before, there are so many options in terms of remedies and, rather than matching a medicine to an illness, it's about matching the medicine to the person. Looking back, there were some clues that we could be looking for a remedy from the sea—her love of water sports, sleeping with a blanket covering her, a dislike of bright light and love (albeit also fear) of the dark could be clues in this direction. Stoi kenti even has dreams of kidnapping as part of the proving! The work that has gone into compiling the resources that we're able to use is amazing; between the proving materials, homeopathic repertories, *Materia Medicas* and programs, they are a true gift to healing for so many.

Two weeks on, I got an update from Bex and her mum. While she'd been able to do more, she'd also developed a sore throat and had a massive eczema eruption that appeared like a lump below her eye. We have a few things we get excited about in homeopathy and someone getting fever-like symptoms can be a great sign that the immune system is responding to a medicine. A return of old symptoms is another potential call for excitement, giving insights that you're on the right track with a well-matching remedy. Bex was doing both here.

When we met for our first follow-up after a month, Bex told me how she was now awake for around ten hours a day. When awake she felt 'normal', where before, she would feel so ill she'd just have some food and go back to bed. The lump below her eye had gone up and down but now was just like a little raised stye-like lump. Bex felt the remedy was definitely making a difference and her mum agreed, recounting that she would hear her singing and knew she must be feeling a lot better. We continued the remedy daily.

Bex and I continued to work together for over two years, meeting at regular intervals, and we continued to see positive progress. Both Bex and her mum had felt the impact of changes from the remedy and, at times, other homeopathic medicines when indicated. Overall, she had increased energy, reduced anxiety, a complete resolution of the eczema, improved sleep and a significant reduction in pain. She was able to do more socially and returned to attending full-time education.

Her progress wasn't always linear—there were times when she slipped back into sleeping more and experiencing more pain, so we altered her homeopathic medicines if needed. The Stoi kenti, in varying potencies, continued to be supportive alongside other medicines for her symptoms. Ultimately, her progress was remarkable, particularly given that her conventional options were limited. Today, she enjoys a typical college student's life, going out and having fun with friends instead of sleeping for hours on end.

I particularly wanted to share this case to demonstrate Bex's patience, persistence and determination that I felt shone through here, which for me has been a big part of working with Bex and her mum. It wasn't always quick or easy, but Bex is now in a far different place than when we first met.

In October 2023, I had a text from her mum to say:

"Would just like to share our good news. Bex started college in September and has not missed a single class. We continued with

Stoi kenti. She is better. She helped move one tonne of logs yesterday after college. She is out today with friends. She went to the cinema last weekend. Everything is going good. But no one believes it's homeopathy, including her grandmother. Absolutely unbelievable. They say it is because she moved schools. Really. I guess I can't have everything. A big thank you from me and her dad and Bex xxxx"

10

ANIMALS

It's vital that I mention in this section that in the UK, you need to be a veterinary surgeon to practice homeopathy with animals.[1] It is illegal for me to prescribe homeopathy for anyone's animals but my own, however, there are some brilliant vets qualified in homeopathy who integrate the two beautifully and I'm grateful this is where my introduction to homeopathy came from.

The cases I share here are examples of using homeopathy with my own animals. You'll recall that my first experience of homeopathy was when John Saxton, a veterinary homeopath, treated our horse, Kara. I'll finish up the Real Life Stories section with three other marvellous instances of using homeopathy with animals—two with my dogs and one again with Kara after she contracted Cushing's disease. This feels like it brings us full circle back to where we began. Here are the last three stories. Thank you for journeying with me!

MıA

Our little re-homed Pug cross Lhasa Apso, Mia, had something going on with her eye and was struggling a little to open it fully. Being a Pug cross, Mia doesn't have the best breeding in terms of eye and nose health but fortunately in general she's in fairly good shape. Her eyes could get some discharge in them at times, but her breathing was far better than stories I've heard about others in her pug-sisterhood.

At first, it looked as if she might have something in her eye, though we couldn't see anything that could be causing the discomfort. I knew if my attempt with a homeopathic remedy didn't help, I'd take her to the vet, especially as there weren't a lot of clues to go on and Mia obviously couldn't give me a description!

The medicine Euphrasia (herbal name 'eyebright') is often a great homeopathic remedy for eye symptoms, though as you've hopefully picked up throughout this text, there are plenty of others. Silica was my other choice, which is brilliant for helping to push out foreign bodies. Indeed, it has achieved a certain fame as the 'number one remedy for splinters'. My daughter opts for taking a few tablets of Silica over my offer to remove a splinter with a sterilised needle every time!

I love single remedy prescribing—it's the mainstay of my practice—but at certain times, I'll give a combined medicine. In this instance I gave Mia both Euphrasia and Silica to cover my bases, putting them inside her cheek. Within twenty seconds, possibly less, her eye was back to normal. It looked to relapse a minute or two later but with one repetition of the remedies, it went away and didn't return. My daughter was there with me and pointed out the speed at which it happened. How wonderful that at times we can help those around us rapidly, effectively and permanently. I love it!

As I write this, it occurred to me that Mia's eyes have remained in far better health since these remedies were taken. Prior to that, they would frequently be 'gunky' and have to be cleaned quite often—it's unfortunately a side effect of a dog breed with slightly bulging eyes. Brachycephalic, or flat-faced, dog breeds like pugs can suffer with this more than other breeds. However, I'm happy to say that Mia's eyes have been much clearer ever since this experience, which is great to recognise.

Lucy

Our lurcher (German Shepherd cross Greyhound), Lucy, was another homeopathic success story in our house, although this case was slightly more challenging than Mia's and much, much messier!

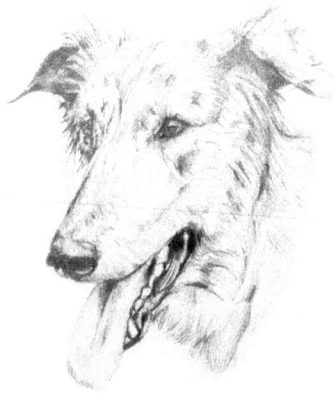

Lucy

Lucy was fourteen weeks old when we picked her up in Liverpool. We were advised to put her in a crate to transport her home and, while I wouldn't do it again, we chose to follow that advice at the time. Whether it was the stress of the crate or of leaving her previous home or the motion of the car, she vomited and had diarrhoea several times on that first journey to our house, and every time after that, when we travelled we had one or the other.

I tried homeopathic medicine after medicine. There are various remedies that are well-known for helping with travel sickness (as ever, where the symptoms fit) such as Cocculus, Tabacum, Nux vomica, Petroleum—and plenty of these felt to fit what was going on, but nothing helped. We also tried feeding her in the car, hanging out and playing in the car to desensitise her around it, travelling with her on my knee or with others sitting next to her in the back seat (which was a little like Russian roulette with a vomit loaded gun!), using ginger essential oil in the boot of the car (we'd been told ginger was good for travel sickness), and feeding her at different times of the day depending on when we were going out in the car. All of it did nothing. At all.

It was while chatting to a homeopathic vet friend about other things that I thought to ask his opinion. It's funny how sometimes you may forget the bigger picture, especially when dealing with your own family. After telling him all we'd done, he asked the most insightful question, 'Who is she as a dog?' Well, of course! Lucy is, or at least appears to be, super joyful. She wants to be friends with everyone, she wants to be near you and—I frequently joke—she has the delusion that everyone loves her. But she could also be easily scared, slightly nervy. When I looked at all of that and included it in my approach, it felt clear that Phosphorus could be a good match, as it also fitted beautifully with her symptoms. I gave her the remedy and finally, success—no more sickness, no more diarrhoea in the car! She also went from being very reticent about getting in the car to being perfectly happy to jump in. The Phosphorus needed repeating only once and we haven't had any issues travelling since. Definitely a joyful change and such a relief for all concerned!

Another beautiful thing—while we gave the remedy for her car sickness, she seemed to take a giant leap forward in terms of her confidence too. Even other dog walkers mentioned it. The difference was huge!

KARA

Our horse had another encounter with homeopathy later in her life that I'd like to share here. Kara had a few bouts of laminitis and we noted that she had grown an unusually thick coat, which wasn't seeming to shed as expected. We sought advice from our local team of horse vets and after further testing, Kara was diagnosed with Cushing's disease.[2] Initially, we went with the conventional vet's advice to give medication to manage her disease. For a period of time, she appeared to tolerate the meds with no side effects but after a year or so, we noticed problems with her gait. She would stagger, almost resembling the walk of a person under the influence of a decent amount of alcohol, and while she shared our taste in an occasional hot chocolate, there was definitely no brandy involved!

I can't tell you why we didn't think to contact the homeopathic vet initially but I can tell you that when she started to respond badly to the medication, that was the first thing we did. We knew who to call this time, and got in touch with veterinary homeopath Brendan Clarke, who by then had taken over the Towerwood veterinary practice in Leeds from John Saxton. Brendan told us about a homeopathic combination remedy that had shown positive results in both horses and dogs with Cushing's disease and suggested we started using that.[3] It was a no-brainer to try the remedy as, at the time, we'd thought Kara might have even had a stroke, based on the symptoms she was presenting, and possibly have to be put down. The idea that it could merely be a side effect of the medication brought us all a ray of hope! Sure enough, stopping the conventional meds and starting the homeopathic combination saw her back to walking normally, with no return of her Cushing's symptoms.

I'll finish this section back where I started on my homeopathy journey, with a quote from homeopathic vet Chris Day. If you remember, Chris was the vet first recommended to my family when we were facing the prospect of having Kara's eye removed. In a short video[4] made for the Faculty of Homeopathy, Chris says about his use of homeopathy in his practice, 'For me, I couldn't be without it because I can do things for animals that I couldn't do any other way. I can help chronic disease in a way that nothing else can. People are always having their animals suffer diseases that are not manageable by conventional medicine and there has to be something else. Quite often, homeopathy happens to be that something else.'

Homeopathy and Lifestyle

It was years ago that I decided to stop consuming alcohol. I remember walking up a hill with Lucy, our lurcher, and feeling worn out. I looked back and wondered if the gin and tonic I'd had the evening before might have had something to do with it, especially as I'd walked up that same hill the day before and handled it just fine. There were a few similar events that happened around the same time and I decided enough was enough and I'd have a year off alcohol. I'm still grateful to my daughter, who bet me that I wouldn't be able to do it. Well, I can resist alcohol easier than I can resist a challenge! I'll be honest and say I've revisited this decision a time or two—a cocktail on holiday, for example—which actually helped me strengthen my resounding feeling that I am healthier and happier without it. My year-long experiment to cut out alcohol was in 2017 and I still think it's been one of my best ever decisions. I believe being alcohol-free has supported me in feeling more alive, more joyful and simply better overall on a day-to-day basis.

Of course, not everyone who uses homeopathy is necessarily going to give up drinking alcohol or occasionally eating foodstuffs that don't entirely suit them, and I certainly don't believe we need to live like saints—I'm definitely nowhere close to that! However,

I do believe our lifestyle has a big part to play in how we feel on a physical, mental and emotional level, and learning to listen to what we need—which can be different for each and every one of us—can be really helpful as we move towards a more joyful, vibrant way of living.

Sometimes, as the quote from homeopathic veterinarian Chris Day says at the end of the last chapter, homeopathy can be the thing that makes all the difference. However, if we're eating unhealthy foods, living a sedentary lifestyle, drinking lots of alcohol, sitting at screens all day, experiencing a lot of stress and not getting enough sleep, then taking a few homeopathic medicines is probably not going to fix everything for us. Sometimes we may need more than one thing to support our health, and how we care for our bodies on a daily basis can help swing the pendulum in the right direction. As I mentioned earlier, the old adage that the best doctors are sunshine, air, exercise, water, diet, rest and laughter gives us a foundation for health that is as old as time. If we are paying attention to these aspects of our lives, it's likely we're setting ourselves up for a healthy body, mind and spirit.

Dr Rangan Chatterjee, in his various books, talks about some key aspects of lifestyle medicine.[1] In his books, as well as in his popular TEDx talk, *'How to make diseases disappear'*,[2] Dr Chatterjee reminds us that getting out in fresh air, exercising and moving our bodies, eating healthily, resting and sleeping well are all great places to start. It seems simple enough, but some of us may struggle to make positive changes. I'm not here to judge. I can definitely be in the camp of not getting enough exercise—I consider myself an expert at 'starting running'—I can get over-excited about work projects and forget to rest as much as I should, and the mind boggles at just how much I would drink in the past, particularly during my student years.

This is another area where I see homeopathy as being so supportive. For example, we all know 'we are what we eat'. Personally, I've found that sugar and plant-based 'teeth-healthy' sweeteners are not head-healthy for me, and carb-rich foods, much as I may love them, love me a bit less. In my practice, I've lost count of the number of clients who feel addicted to a certain food—they have a feeling of not being able to do without something even though they know it's not helping them—but after a well-matched remedy, they frequently tell me they no longer have the craving. As we choose to move towards a greater state of health, homeopathy can be a good place to start. Not only can it help remove symptoms that cause us to feel ill, but there is something about homeopathy that often allows those who use it to find more ease, balance and harmony overall.

We all have to do what makes sense for us and it helps to remember that we are not static beings—what may have supported us at one time in our lives might not do the trick now, and what works for one person might not work for another. Yet at any stage, homeopathy can potentially contribute to a greater sense of wellness. In thinking back to Sarah, who you read about in the Mental Health section of our real life stories, she took anti-depressants for a long time until she decided she wanted to try another option. I love that she was able to work with homeopathy *and* her GP to reduce her meds and ultimately feel happier, healthier and more present all around. In Sarah's words:

> *"I experienced something that I'd never experienced before in my life—a real sense of contentment and inner resilience and a real sense that the world was okay, that I had the skills to deal with it, and that things stopped fazing me."*

Closing Thoughts

There is an acronym in the medical world—TEETH—'Tried Everything Else, Try Homeopathy'.[1] As humorous as this may sound, it belies the truth of the matter—that homeopathy is in fact one of the most effective medicines we have at our disposal for treating all manner of ailments. I would argue that, far from it being the last thing to try, homeopathy could, in many cases, be one of the first.

Some time ago, I asked a number of people who had experienced homeopathic treatment to describe homeopathy in one word. Re-reading these words makes me smile. Here are some of the expressions they came up with:

**Life-changing | Life-saving | Power to self-heal
Miraculous | Empowering | No-brainer | A blessing
Freedom | Personalised | Individualised**

I then asked what kinds of conditions homeopathy had helped them with:

**Depression | Anxiety | Hay fever | Ear infections
Stammering | Pre-menopausal symptoms | Allergies**

Irregular menses | Colitis | Complex PTSD
Autoimmune illnesses

You'll notice that this list mentions a fairly wide range of conditions that includes not only physical, but mental and emotional symptoms too, and gives us a small insight into the substantial scope of homeopathy.

'Magic' is a word I often hear my clients use when describing the results of their homeopathic treatments, and it's used in more than one of the stories shared in this book. When my daughter was younger, she and I used to call homeopathic medicines 'magic tablets' and I've lost count of the number of times someone has referred to seeing changes following homeopathy as 'like magic'.

I know not everyone is comfortable using this word. In 2017, my friend and colleague Ananda More produced a film called *Magic Pills*.[2] The film's title caused quite a stir and I was intrigued by how frequently Ananda was questioned by people in the homeopathic community about her use of 'the M-word'. Granted, our discomfort may have something to do with homeopathic practitioners being called 'snake oil salesmen' and the practice labelled 'pseudoscience' over the years. Some make a connection with witchcraft or magic tricks. I have a feeling that historically many of us with nature-loving tendencies, especially those working with healing modalities, might have been burnt at the stake. I can see how a simple five-letter word could carry a gravitas beyond its mere letters.

I can appreciate why some people get upset by the word, why some are intrigued by it and why others love it. We're all different and it would be foolish to expect those in a profession which is built on individuality to all think the same. Personally, I'm happy to embrace the mysterious, the unexplained, the 'magic' in the everyday. While I know there's a scientific explanation behind the sunrise and the sunset, how the waves swell and the tides work, it doesn't feel any less amazing when I'm experiencing them. I feel a joy and magic in each.

With a well-matched homeopathic remedy, the changes that I see can feel magical—even impossible—sometimes and, as you've read in the stories in this book, sometimes we are told those changes *are* impossible. Yet I get to witness them happen. With the level of research being conducted today, there may be a 'how' coming soon, but for now, I'm more than happy to celebrate the unexplainable. Perhaps it's *because* of the unexplainable nature of homeopathy that over the years the practice has attracted so much opposition and even at times, downright hostility.

I want to be honest here. If you were to ask me as a homeopath if I can help you, my response would be 'I don't know'. The only thing I can guarantee is that I'll do my best. I often describe myself as impatient. I want people to get better as soon as possible because I don't want anyone to suffer, so I work hard to help people where I can. While I've seen amazing things happen, some of which I've written about in these pages, I don't always see the kinds of successes I've described in this book. It's relatively rare that I don't see positive changes but it does happen. Sometimes homeopathy isn't right for what a person needs at that stage. Sometimes the remedy given wasn't quite the right match and we needed more time. Sometimes *I'm* not the right match for a client who walked in the door. Sometimes it's something else altogether that's going on. One of the joys of having different modalities and practitioners is that, if I'm not the right person, the chances are that either working with someone else or using a different approach may well help with the symptoms someone is struggling with. The ways in which we personally define success, interact with the world and respond to a system of medicine can be as varied as the homeopathic medicines we use. This is as it should be—we are all unique individuals.

During the time I was writing this book, I attended a teaching seminar with Drs Bhawisha and Shachindra Joshi. Listening to their shared wisdom regarding their work in clinic, Bhawisha said, 'Shachindra and I have learnt from our successes but we have learnt much more from our mistakes or failures.' That goes for me too. I think it's actually a good rule of thumb in work, and in life. When we learn from our mistakes and failures, ultimately, we have not truly failed. I know I'm here for the long run. I will continue to walk alongside anyone who might like me to. And I'm as grateful for those I've witnessed get better as I am for the lessons I've learned from those who haven't.

While I can't help everyone or change everything, I've come to know over time that homeopathy is highly effective. I wouldn't be doing what I do otherwise. I've certainly been intrigued by other systems, but I always come back to the fact that homeopathy is the most inclusive, individualised and effective form of supporting people that I've found.

There are homeopaths all over the world seeing beautiful changes for people, like the ones you've learned about in this book. There are hundreds of experiences shared daily on social media and I've shared plenty like them myself. This book is just a small insight into the potential of homeopathy. Watch the films, listen to podcasts, follow homeopaths on social media, read some of the texts about why people became homeopaths—there are so many inspiring stories out there!

It also feels important that I mention there are many ways to practise and use homeopathy. This book represents an insight into my work—other practitioners may well work differently. Years ago, when our horse was treated for her eye disease, I discussed this with a friend at school. I told her about the one tablet a day for five days approach we'd been recommended. She said, 'That's not how you do homeopathy,' and went on to share how it had been suggested she take her remedy. For her, it was using a homeopathic medicine in water which she diluted several times and then took a spoonful of the diluted mix. I'm happy to say they're both perfectly good ways of using homeopathy and, as you've read, our experience with it was highly effective. I sometimes give remedies as a dry dose and sometimes as a liquid dose—they are both homeopathy! I've also shared some insights into frequency of taking the medicines—again, not everyone works like I do and that's all good too. As you've read, our aim is to work with the individual in front of us and match the medicine and the potency to their symptoms and energy.

Of course, as I've said before, I'm also a fan of working with other modalities alongside homeopathy. In my own joyful health journey, particularly around my headaches and migraines, it was a combination of things that worked for me and it wasn't a quick fix. Finding a homeopathic medicine that really suited me was a bit of a mission. The remedy I ended up with is one of our rarer ones (it still hasn't made it into the repertories yet); it took working with a homeopath, and quite some time, before I got there in the end. In addition to homeopathy, lifestyle changes, massage, physiotherapy and dietary changes all played a key part. Fitting these various elements together for myself has taken time, but I'm very grateful for the learning along the way. It's important to do what makes sense to you.

As I conclude my journey of writing this book, I end where I began, with the **joys** of doing the work that I'm very grateful I do. There are many:

There is a great deal of **joy in listening** as someone shares who they are and how they experience life. It is a privilege rarely afforded in the outside world and I get to experience it almost every day. While I can't predict the future or control outcomes, I see you as a person, hear you and offer homeopathy as a potential catalyst for change.

There is **joy in being a witness to healing**. The word 'healing' means 'restoration to health' or 'restoration to wholeness'. People who experience the benefits of homeopathy often tell me things like, 'I feel more like me', 'I feel more in balance' or 'I feel more present'. This is part of what we're aiming for. I am often a witness for the changes that result when someone experiences a well-matching homeopathic medicine. It is an incredible privilege to do this work.

There is **joy in learning**. For me, this is a big one. I would definitely say I was one of the geekier kids at school (a pair of big 1980s specs helped to seal the deal) and learning was always a happy place for me. Now, I am absolutely a 'homeopathy geek'. As I study the energies of our medicines, I'm learning about the energies of plants, minerals and animals that also call our planet home. It is incredibly joyful, satisfying and awe-inspiring.

There is **joy in learning from the inspirational people** who have traversed this path before and with me. The brilliant work that has gone into refining and developing this system of medicine is extraordinary. We are truly standing on the shoulders of giants. The repertories, books, proving data, research and clinical experience that I can readily access and use to help myself and others restore health fills me with so much gratitude, as do those who are continuing the work as you read this.

I find **joy in collaborating with other practitioners**. As I've said before, while homeopathy has proven to be amazing, I don't believe there is any one system that can do everything. As a result, this keeps me on my toes, sends me off to learn more, leads me to new discoveries and opens me up to recommending and working with other experts in their chosen fields.

I've found great **joy in the connections** my work has brought me. Most people come to me because someone else has suggested they try homeopathy. It might be someone I've seen in clinic or a friend or acquaintance who has had success working with another practitioner. I've had clients referred to me by swimming teachers, pharmacists, nurses, friends, family members, parents picking their children up from lessons, other homeopaths and holistic practitioners and more. This work has brought amazing colleagues, fabulous friends and awe-inspiring experiences that I could never have imagined. Who would I be without all that? It's all been remarkable and I am eternally grateful.

While I'm not particularly religious, I do feel that there is a bigger force at work. Before I start a clinic session, I often offer up a prayer that I am able to help this person to the best of my ability. It wasn't until I read Marianne Williamson's *A Return to Love* that I realised there are many names for this universal energy. Earlier in my life, I struggled with the whole 'white man in sandals' concept of God as it was presented to me, but now I get joy from my feeling that none of us are alone, that we are supported by something (no matter what we call it) and perhaps it is this that is leading us to our wholeness, to our healing journey of self-discovery and more. 'Know thyself'—a quote attributed to Plato—feels significant here. In working with homeopathy, I've come to understand and know myself better and I've seen many others do the same.

Finally, I hope the stories I've shared in this book have come alive for you. I hope I've allowed the potential of homeopathy as an incredible system of medicine to shine through. And I hope you have found the level of joy in reading these pages that I have found in writing them.

I wish you health, happiness and joy,

Acknowledgements

We wouldn't be talking about homeopathy without the work of Dr Samuel Hahnemann, who first mentioned the word in an essay in 1796 and devoted the rest of his life to developing the art and science of it. I have eternal gratitude to him and those who followed afterwards for the work they tirelessly pursued, and to so many for following his path.

Other influential teachers and mentors include Dr Annette Sneevliet, Drs Bhawisha and Shachindra Joshi, along with Grazia Gatti, Helen Dalton and Ilana Dannheisser, who so passionately share the Joshis' work with us here in the UK and beyond. Helen sadly died in 2022 but her teachings (and incredible sense of style) will be remembered by many of us for a long time. I love listening to the teachings of veterinary homeopath Geoff Johnson and Dr Jonathon Hardy too. Also Dr Rajan Sankaran, whose work I have touched on and feel am still to dive into more fully. His phrase 'the non-human song' is something that resonates deeply with me.

I want to thank Jackie McTaggart, who shared so generously her understanding of Dr Jan Scholten's work with myself and colleagues for several years after I graduated from the North West College of Homeopathy. Scholten has been a constant inspiration throughout my practice, and I have huge amounts of gratitude for the work he's done on the Periodic Table (and since with the plants in homeopathy), as well as everyone at the college who gave me the foundation to go forth and grow from there.

I don't think this book would exist without the teachings of Jeremy Sherr in his Dynamis course.[1] It was this course and the people I met on it that encouraged me to step out of my quiet country mouse life. When I teach or supervise students, I find myself quoting Jeremy frequently. His wisdom is in my heart and I am grateful to be able to share his gems with others.

My journey with homeopathy for myself started with meeting Sue Asquith, my first homeopath. If I can embody a little of how she worked—with empathy, wisdom, a passion for homeopathy and some great knowledge, then I'll be very happy. It was Sue who said, with curiosity, at one of our consultations, 'Why aren't you doing homeopathy?'—a beautiful catalyst to my journey here today. For being an absolute inspiration, and everything else, I am truly grateful.

I am also immensely grateful to my past and current supervisors, who are all fabulous, and in particular Andrene, who has listened to me talk about this book, encouraged my writing of it and also urged me to rest—something I often forget to do between my excitement and joy about life.

I'm grateful to the people who first trusted and emboldened me to teach, to give back to students some of what I'd learnt along the way. It was Andrene and Rachael—at the North West College of Homeopathy—who asked me to give a lecture called 'The Joy of Practice' in 2023, which sparked the title of this book. Andrene told me, 'We chose the title specifically for you to weave your sparkle into the group so that they can see the joy to be gained from becoming a homeopath and going into practice.' I am fortunate to teach at several homeopathy colleges where there are some seriously brilliant students rising through the ranks. They teach me so much and I am excited to see them step out into practice.

There are people working tirelessly on homeopathy research—in laboratories, in clinics, on publications and much more. Then there are the people making a leap of faith—pharmacists who recommend homeopathy, teachers and lecturers who spread the message with passion, and doctors, who, despite being told time and again it's nonsense, continue to pursue homeopathy and seek help when the mainstream world fails to acknowledge it. There are so many professionals who contribute to the work we do in clinic every day. I thank you all.

My daughter Isla and my partner Steve, whose stories both feature in this book, are a complete inspiration to me. I wouldn't be who I am today without either of them. That also goes for my parents, Sue and Roy, and my sister, Ruth, who have always supported and believed in me consistently, tirelessly and compassionately. Also my sister-in-law, Lel, a talented graphic designer who took my ideas for the cover and turned them into something better than I could ever have imagined.

Friends who've encouraged me—your support was bigger than you may realise and, on some days when I was driving myself crazy editing, I would remember your encouraging comments or conversations, which would remind me why I was doing this project!

A huge thank you goes to the people—primarily my clients, but also friends and family—who were willing to allow me to share their stories in this book. In some cases the names have been changed for privacy reasons but for those who wished their real names to appear, I have honoured that.

I need to thank Helen Strong and Bold Fish Publishing. Without Helen, this book would be far more rambling with much more waffle—she has taken my offering and helped me craft it into an accessible format, while being a supportive mentor along the way. Also, Julie Trager, who came on board as an editor a few months into the process, has been amazing to work with—another gift of creating this book. Thanks too to Enya Marczak and Olivia Marczak for the plant and animal sketches which appear throughout the book, and for putting up with my 'just one more last change' requests!

To all the people who have read my manuscript and offered suggestions of edits, inclusions, amendments and endorsements, I have huge gratitude to all of you. Any mistakes are mine.

Last, but certainly not least, thank you to you, the reader, for taking the time to engage with the stories here. Without the tales and accounts of my clients, and without you reading them, this book would merely be me speaking into an endless vacuum.

Homeopathy truly is an incredible profession to be involved in and I am grateful to everyone who has influenced my path to where I am today.

Notes

Introduction

1. 5ft 7in or 177m tall at her shoulder

Some Homeopathic Terminology

1. www.collinsdictionary.com/dictionary/english/polychrest

2. www.emmacolley.co.uk/blog/potencies-in-homeopathy

3. www.emmacolley.co.uk/blog/strange-rare-and-peculiar-symptoms

4. hpathy.com/pharmacology/trituration-succussion-history-medicine

What Is Homeopathy?

1. www.etymonline.com/word/homeopathy

2. Full name Philippus Aureolus Theophrastus Bombastus von Hohenheim b. 1493, Einsiedeln, Switzerland, d. 1541

3. www.homeobook.com/paracelsus-and-homoeopathy

4. www.homeopathyschool.com/the-school/editorial/the-organon/aphorism-1-10

5. www.phrases.org.uk/meanings/less-is-more.html

6. The full quote is, 'All things are poison, and nothing is without poison; the dosage alone makes it so a thing is not a poison.' en.wikipedia.org/wiki/The_dose_makes_the_poison

7. www.ncbi.nlm.nih.gov/pmc/articles/PMC1297514

8. www.thelancet.com/journals/lancet/article/PIIS0140-6736(22)00088-5/fulltext

Homeopathy and Conventional Medicine

1. drchatterjee.com

2. www.nutritank.com

3. youtu.be/pe0_tYhTxgQ

4. medical-dictionary.thefreedictionary.com/placebo+effect

5. www.ncbi.nlm.nih.gov/pmc/articles/PMC8488027

6. www.ncbi.nlm.nih.gov/pmc/articles/PMC3181672

7. pubmed.ncbi.nlm.nih.gov/16296912

8. pubmed.ncbi.nlm.nih.gov/19135953

9. www.ncbi.nlm.nih.gov/pmc/articles/PMC5600367

10. www.researchgate.net/publication/7709477_Outcome_and_costs_of_
homoeopathic_and_conventional_treatment_strategies_A_comparative_cohort_
study_in_patients_with_chronic_disorders

11. www.etymonline.com/search?q=healing

12. www.emmacolley.co.uk/homeopathy-and-wikipedia.html

13. organonofmedicine.com

14. www.hahnemannhouse.org/constantine-hering-and-homeopathy

15. hpathy.com/organon-philosophy/herings-law-of-direction-of-cure-a-reliable-tool-
in-homeopathic-therapeutics

16. archive.org/details/materiamedicapu00dudggoog

17. pubmed.ncbi.nlm.nih.gov/24200828

18. homeopathy-uk.org/treatment/scientific-evidence-and-homeopathy

1. Headaches and Migraines

1. www.lancaster.ac.uk/news/articles/2018/86-million-workdays-lost-to-migraine-
in-the-uk-every-year

2. Respiratory Issues

1. Established in the UK in 1996 by David Needleman, the HomeopathicHelpline offers immediate assistance and acute advice to patients who are unable to contact their usual practitioner. It is also a valuable resource to other healthcare professionals. The website is www.thehomeopathichelpline.com and the telephone service at 09065 343404 operates from 9:00a.m. to midnight every day of the year.

2. www.facultyofhomeopathy.org/pages/dr-jonathan-hardy

4. Skin Complaints
1. hpathy.com/homeopathy-papers/what-you-can-expect-after-taking-a-remedy
2. hpathy.com/organon-philosophy/herings-law-of-direction-of-cure-a-reliable-tool-in-homeopathic-therapeutics

5. Women's Health
1. www.glucosegoddess.com

6. Arthritis and Joint Complaints
1. www.nhs.uk/conditions/rheumatoid-arthritis/causes
2. www.nice.org.uk/guidance/ng100/resources/rheumatoid-arthritis-in-adults-management-pdf-66141531233989

7. Mental Health
1. www.psychologytoday.com/us/blog/psychiatry-through-the-looking-glass/202108/are-children-and-adolescents-overprescribed
2. www.cchrint.org/psychiatric-drugs/children-on-psychiatric-drugs
3. www.nhsbsa.nhs.uk/statistical-collections/medicines-used-mental-health-england/medicines-used-mental-health-england-201516-202223

8. Mulitple Issues
1. www.webmd.com/covid/what-are-covid-toes

9. Managing Side Effects
1. link.springer.com/article/10.1007/s00238-019-01618-7
2. The Medicines Healthcare Regulatory Authority (MHRA) states: 'All vaccines and medicines have some side effects although not everybody gets them. These side effects need to be continuously balanced against the expected benefits in preventing illness.'
www.gov.uk/government/publications/coronavirus-covid-19-vaccine-adverse-reactions/coronavirus-vaccine-summary-of-yellow-card-reporting
3. From the MHRA website: 'It is estimated that only 10% of serious reactions and between 2 and 4% of non-serious reactions are reported. Under-reporting coupled with a decline in reporting makes it especially important to report all suspicions of adverse drug reactions to the Yellow Card Scheme.'
www.gov.uk/drug-safety-update/yellow-card-please-help-to-reverse-the-decline-in-

reporting-of-suspected-adverse-drug-reactions

4. Postural orthostatic tachycardia syndrome (POTS) is one of a group of disorders that have orthostatic intolerance (OI) as their primary symptom. OI is a condition in which an excessively reduced volume of blood returns to the heart after an individual stands up from a lying down position. www.ninds.nih.gov/health-information/disorders/postural-tachycardia-syndrome-pots

5. www.gov.uk/government/publications/freedom-of-information-responses-from-the-mhra-week-commencing-22-february-2021/foi-21132-reported-side-effect-data-for-vaccinations-6-in-1-rotavirus-men-b-pneumococcal-hibmen-c-mmr-flu-spray-and-injection-and-4-in-1

10. Animals

1. Veterinary surgeons will have MRCVS (Member of the Royal College of Veterinary Surgeons) or FRCVS (Fellow of the Royal College of Veterinary Surgeons) after their name. Those who have additionally qualified as homeopathic vets will also have VetMF-Hom (Veterinary Member of the Faculty of Homeopathy) or VetFFHom (Veterinary Fellow of the Faculty of Homeopathy) after this.

2. www.rvc.ac.uk/equine-vet/information-and-advice/fact-files/cushings-disease

3. pubmed.ncbi.nlm.nih.gov/11212087PR

4. youtu.be/6B5OK0cjIJI

Homeopathy and Lifestyle

1. drchatterjee.com

2. youtu.be/gaY4m00wXpw

Closing Thoughts

1. www.allacronyms.com/TEETH/medical

2. magicpillsmovie.com

Acknowledgements

1. www.dynamis.edu

USEFUL RESOURCES

BOOKS

Get Well Soon by **Misha Norland and Mani Norland**
One of the easiest-to-access first aid beginner's homeopathy books I've encountered. Delightfully illustrated and brilliantly described, it's accessible and a great place to start.

Homeopathic Prescribing by **Steven B Kayne and Lee Kayne**
Includes an introduction to using homeopathy for minor ailments and fifty-six handy flowcharts helping to discern what medicine will be suitable in various complaints.

The Practical Handbook of Homoeopathy: The How, When, Why and Which of Home Prescribing by **Colin Griffith**
Described by the publishers at Penguin Random House as 'This user-friendly resource holds authoritative, accessible advice on home prescribing—all you need to understand the How, When and Which of Homoeopathy.'

The Complete Homeopathy Handbook: A Guide to Everyday Health Care by **Miranda Castro**
This was the first homeopathy book I owned and stands the test of time. Castro shares insights into remedies, how to use a basic repertory grid and, alongside homeopathy, offers other alternative health solutions that people may wish to use. Also Castro's *Homeopathy for Pregnancy, Birth and Your Baby's First Year* supported me through pregnancy and baby times.

Pregnancy and Childbirth with Homeopathy by **Gudny Osk Didriksdottir**
A clear, concise guide to supporting health with homeopathy through pregnancy and birth.

Magic of the Minimum Dose and *More Magic of the Minimum Dose* by **Dr Dorothy Shepherd**
Described as 'case histories by a world famous homeopathic doctor', both books are crammed with cases from the early to mid-1900s.

Homoeopathy: A Rational Choice in Medicine by **Mo Morrish**
This book offers a clear and simple overview of homeopathic medicine and the principles which underpin it, along with evidence to support its effectiveness and safety. More than this, it places homeopathy on a level playing field with modern mainstream medicine, dispelling myths and providing a realistic perspective on the two systems of healthcare.

A Homeopathic Love Story by **Rima Handley**
A beautiful insight into Hahnemann's world, this story details the romance between him and his last wife Melanie, along with a greater awareness of medicine at the time and a glimpse into cases treated by Hahnemann himself.

Homeopathy: Medicine for the New Millennium by George Vithouklas

One of the first books I read on the topic, and a fascinating discussion of homeopathy and its place in our world. It presents both 'the historical scientific basis for the discipline in simple terms, and shows that homeopathy not only addresses the health of the whole person, but can succeed in treating many chronic conditions regarded as incurable by conventional medicine.'

The Organon of Medicine by Dr Samuel Hahnemann

The Organon is an incredible text, and there are various translations. Not so much a book for the beginner, for folks passionate about homeopathy it's an in-depth and brilliant book. For those studying homeopathy, it's a must-read.

Lectures on Organon of Medicine by Dr Manish Bhatia

A three-book series, this has been my favourite for a long time.

At the time of writing, Jeremy Sherr is currently finishing writing his Organon book. This will be well worth a read for those interested in exploring *The Organon of Medicine* further.

FILMS

Introducing Homeopathy (2024)

This film premiered at the Joint American Homeopathic Conference in April 2024. At the time of writing, they're aiming for widespread availability on a streaming platform. The website says, '*Introducing Homeopathy* is a new professionally produced, feature-length film dedicated to bringing homeopathy into every household and healthcare system globally.'
introducinghomeopathy.com

Magic Pills by Ananda More (2017)
An inspiring and engaging film examining the evidence behind homeopathy. Featuring researchers from within the homeopathy world and outside of it, the film illustrates projects in Cuba, India, Tanzania and Australia and asks the question, 'Is homeopathy a miracle medicine that can save lives, or is it one of the greatest and most elaborate frauds known to man?'
www.magicpillsmovie.com

Just One Drop by Laurel Chiten (2017)
Released around the same time as _Magic Pills,_ both films take their own unique look at the questions that arise around homeopathy. The _Just One Drop_ website says, 'The film explores the controversy, dispels myths and misconceptions, and asks whether or not homeopathy has been given a fair shake.'
www.justonedropfilm.com

HOMEOPATHIC PHARMACIES

Ainsworth's: www.ainsworths.com
Freeman's Homeopathic Pharmacy: www.freemans.scot
Helios Homoeopathy: www.helios.co.uk
Nelsons: www.nelsonspharmacy.com

USEFUL WEBSITES

Find a Homeopath is the website of 4Homeopathy, who represent ten of the major organisations of homeopathy in the UK. There is a search function to locate homeopaths in your area, as well as lots of information around homeopathy in general.
www.findahomeopath.org

British Homeopathic Dental Association—a group of dentists and dental care professionals that have an interest in using homeopathy alongside dentistry. www.bhda.co.uk

Faculty of Homeopathy—Faculty members are qualified and trained in both conventional medicine and homeopathic medicine. www.facultyofhomeopathy.org

British Homeopathic Veterinary Surgeons—the place to go to find a UK vet practising homeopathy. www.bahvs.net

Homeopathy UK—the UK's leading homeopathic charity. Lots of information around homeopathy, details of charity clinics and more. www.homeopathy-uk.org

If you're outside the UK, the chances are there is a homeopathic or membership organisation where you are. It may be worth contacting them to find out details of locally practising homeopaths.

Homeopathy Training—should you wish to find out more about training to become a homeopath in the UK. www.homeopathytraining.uk

Homeopathy Research Institute—a UK-based charity dedicated to promoting high quality research in homeopathy. www.hri-research.org

Clil Botanicals—created by Camilla Sherr, Co-Founding Director of *Homoeopathy for Health in Africa*, and colleague Michal Agami. Their philosophy is to treat oily skin with oils ('like with like'). They sell cleansing, facial and remedial oils, as well as powerful serums which leave skin healthy, happy and glowing. www.clil-botanicals.com

INDEX

About the Author

After ten years believing she wanted to be a vet, Em Colley realised it was actually working with people, not animals, that she was most intrigued by. To that end, she earned a degree in Psychology and Neuroscience at Manchester University and alongside this, became accredited in Reiki and Reflexology, which were her first steps into the world of alternative medicine.

Em later returned to Manchester to study at the North West College of Homeopathy and has been studying ever since! Graduating as a professional homeopath in 2007, she is as fascinated and excited by the potential of homeopathy as the day she entered into it. She is passionate about sharing the benefits of this amazing system, and loves her work in clinic (consulting both online and in person), as well as teaching at several colleges in the UK and working with supervision with both homeopathy students and practitioners.

Em loves to hang out with her family, including their cat and two dogs, and enjoys creating—crochet, painting stones and writing are currently high on the list. She also enjoys paddle-boarding and walking, and is always reading and learning. While running is an aspiration, she is brilliant at falling out of the habit, recognising that for her, it's perhaps more accurate to call it 'starting running'.

Em can be contacted via her website:
www.emmacolley.co.uk

www.ingramcontent.com/pod-product-compliance
Lightning Source LLC
Chambersburg PA
CBHW031125020426